# Psychiatric-Mental Health Nursing Review and Resource Manual

## 2nd Edition

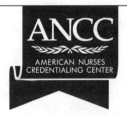

ANCC
AMERICAN NURSES
CREDENTIALING CENTER

Published by:    American Nurses Credentialing Center
Institute for Credentialing Innovation
8515 Georgia Avenue, Suite 400
Silver Spring, MD    20910-3492
www.nursecredentialing.org

ISBN-13:  978-0-9768213-7-3
ISBN-10:  0-9768213-7-0

# Psychiatric-Mental Health Nursing Review and Resource Manual, 2nd Edition

**August 2006**

Please direct your comments and/or queries to:
revmanuals@ana.org

The health care services delivery system is a volatile marketplace demanding superior knowledge, clinical skills, and competencies from all registered nurses. Nursing autonomy of practice and nurse career marketability and mobility in the new century hinge on affirming the profession's formative philosophy, which places a priority on lifelong commitment to the principles of education and professional development. The knowledge base of nursing theory and practice is expanding, and while care has been taken to ensure the accuracy and timeliness of the information presented in this second edition of the *Psychiatric-Mental Health Nursing Review and Resource Manual,* clinicians are advised to always verify the most current national treatment guidelines and recommendations, and to practice in accordance with professional standards of care with regard to the unique circumstances that apply in each practice situation. In addition, every effort has been made in this text to ensure accuracy and, in particular, to confirm that drug selections and dosages are in accordance with current recommendations and practice, including the ongoing research, changes in government regulations, and the developments in product information provided by pharmaceutical manufacturers. However, it is the responsibility of each nurse to verify all information and to practice in accordance with professional standards of care. In addition, the editors wish to note that provision of information in this text does not imply an endorsement of any particular procedures or services.

Therefore, the authors, editors, American Nurses Association (ANA), American Nurses Publishing (ANP), American Nurses Credentialing Center (ANCC), and the Institute for Credentialing Innovation cannot accept responsibility for errors or omissions, or for any consequences or liability, injury and/or damages to persons or property from application of the information in this manual and make no warranty, express or implied, with respect to the contents of the *Psychiatric-Mental Health Nursing Review and Resource Manual, 2nd Ed.*

# Introduction to the Continuing Education (CE) Contact Hour Application Process for *Psychiatric-Mental Health Nursing Review and Resource Manual, 2nd Edition*

The Institute for Credentialing Innovation now offers the continuing education contact hours for this manual online at www.NursingWorld.org, the American Nurses Association's Web site. This process involves answering approximately 50 questions that test knowledge of the information contained within this manual. The continuing education contact hours can be completed at any time and a certificate can be printed from the Web site immediately upon successful completion of the test.

The *Psychiatric-Mental Health Nursing Review and Resource Manual, 2nd Edition,* is designed to meet the following objectives:

1. Identify the major components of the psychiatric evaluation process.

2. Discuss the nurse and clinical nurse specialist's role in the care of patients with psychiatric/mental health disorders.

Upon completion of this manual <u>and</u> the online CE test, a nurse can receive a total of 15 (fifteen) continuing education contact hours. **The entire process—online test and evaluation form—must be completed by December 31, 2008 in order to receive credit.**

To begin the process, please e-mail revmanuals@ana.org *or* go to the ANCC website at www.nursecredentialing.org for specific instructions.

Your patience with this new process is greatly appreciated.

## Inquiries or Comments

If you have any questions about the CE contact hours, please e-mail The Institute at: revmanuals@ana.org. You may also mail any comments to the Editor/Project Manager, at the address listed below.

## Duplicate CE Certificates

Once you have successfully passed the CE test on NursingWorld, you may go back and re-print your certificate as often as you wish.

The Institute for Credentialing Innovation
American Nurses Credentialing Center
Attn: Editor/Project Manager
8515 Georgia Avenue, Suite 400
Silver Spring, MD 20910-3492
Fax: (301) 628-5342

# Introduction

The *Psychiatric Mental Health Nursing Review and Resource Manual, 2nd Ed.,* is designed to help the Psychiatric Mental Health Nurse or the Clinical Nurse Specialist in Psychiatric Mental Health Nursing prepare for the national certification. This manual is the combination of two review manuals with the first section on adult psychiatric mental health nursing and the second section on the child/adolescent psychiatric mental health nursing.

The content discusses the scope and standards of practice of both the advance practice clinical nurse specialist and the psychiatric mental health nurse. This manual addresses the role of the Psychiatric Mental Health nurse and the legal responsibilities that are vital in caring for the psychiatric patient/client. After reviewing the many psychotherapeutic theories, the manual discusses various disorders, the assessment and diagnosis of diseases and appropriate treatment modalities.

The American Nurses Credentialing Center would like to acknowledge the authors who assisted in the development of the first edition of the *Psychiatric-Mental Health Nursing Review and Resource Manual.*

Lorraine Flint Rother, RN, MS, CNS
Beth Good, MSN, CARN, CNS
Mildred Pluim, RN, PhD, CNS
Ann Baker, MA, RNC

# Contents

Contents

# section one

## Adult Psychiatric-Mental Health Nursing

# Nursing Standards, Theories, and Roles

## Nursing Standards

*Code of Ethics for Nurses with Interpretive Statements (2001)*

The American Nurses Association's (ANA) Code of Ethics for Nurses with Interpretive Statements (2001) is a series of written proclamations that describe ideal behaviors and professional attributes for nurses. The Code provides a framework for nurses to guide their nursing judgments and decision-making. See Table 1-1.

---

*Table 1-1 Proclamations of ANA's Code of Ethics for Nurses with Interpretive Statements*

---

1  The nurse, in all professional relationships, practices with compassion and respect for the inherent dignity, worth and uniqueness of every individual, unrestricted by considerations of social or economic status, personal attributes, or the nature of health problems.

2  The nurse's primary commitment is to the patient, whether an individual, family, group or community.

3  The nurse promotes, advocates for and strives to protect the health, safety and rights of the patient.

4  The nurse is responsible and accountable for individual nursing practice and determines the appropriate delegation of tasks consistent with the nurse's obligation to provide optimum patient care.

5  The nurse owes the same duties to self as to others, including the responsibility to preserve integrity and safety, to maintain competence and to continue personal and professional growth.

6  The nurse participates in establishing, maintaining and improving healthcare environments and conditions of employment conducive to the provision of quality healthcare and consistent with the values of the profession through individual and collective action.

*Continued on page 2*

*Table 1-1, continued*

7 The nurse participates in the advancement of the profession through contributions to practice, education, administration, and knowledge development.

8 The nurse collaborates with other health professionals and the public in promoting community, national, and international efforts to meet health needs.

9 The profession of nursing, as represented by associations and their members, is responsible for articulating nursing values, for maintaining the integrity of the profession and its practice and for shaping social policy.

©2001 American Nurses Association. Reprinted with permission. American Nurses Association.

## Nursing's Social Policy Statement (American Nurses Association, 2003)

*Nursing's Social Policy Statement* is a document that nurses can use as a framework for understanding nursing's relationships with society and nursing's obligation to those who receive nursing care. Nursing is dynamic, rather than static, and reflects the changing nature of societal need. See Table 1-2.

*Table 1-2 Selected Statements, Nursing's Social Policy Statement*

*Underlying Values and Assumptions*
• Humans manifest an essential unity of mind/ body/spirit.

• Human experience is contextually and culturally defined.

• Health and illness are human experiences.

• The presence of illness does not preclude health nor does optimal health preclude illness.

*Essential Features of Professional Nursing*
• Attention to the full range of human experiences and responses to health and illness without restriction to a problem-focused orientation

• Integration of objective data with knowledge gained from an understanding of the patient or group's subjective experience

• Application of scientific knowledge to the processes of diagnosis and treatment

• Provision of a caring relationship that facilitates health and healing

©2003 American Nurses Association. Reprinted with permission. American Nurses Association

## Scope and Standards of Psychiatric-Mental Health Nursing Practice (American Nurses Association, 2000)

### Levels of Practice

Psychiatric-mental health nurses are qualified to practice nursing at two levels—basic and advanced. The levels of practice are differentiated by educational preparation, practice complexity, and skill to perform certain nursing functions (Society for Education and Research for Psychiatric-Mental Health Nursing, 1996).

### Basic Level

The registered nurse who practices in psychiatric-mental health nursing at the basic level has received a baccalaureate degree in nursing, has provided practice in the field of psychiatric-mental health nursing for a minimum of two years, and demonstrates the skills necessary as outlined in the *Scope and Standards of Psychiatric-Mental Health Nursing Practice* (2000) document.

Basic-level practice includes such nursing tasks as:
- using interventions to foster and promote optimal mental health,
- assessing dysfunction,
- assisting patients in regaining or improving their coping abilities,
- maximizing their strengths, and
- preventing further disability.

Additional tasks include:
- administering and monitoring psychobiological treatment regimens (e.g., prescribed psychopharmacological medications and their effects),
- assisting and monitoring patients in self-care activities,
- case management, counseling, and crisis care,
- health maintenance and health promotion,
- health teaching,
- intake screenings, evaluation,
- milieu therapy (providing a therapeutic environment), and
- psychiatric rehabilitation.

### Advanced Level

The advanced practice psychiatric-mental health nurse (APRN-PMH) is a licensed RN, educationally prepared at the master's level, and nationally certified as a clinical specialist in psychiatric-mental health nursing. The APRN-PMH is distinguished by the depth of knowledge of theory and practice, substantiated experience in clinical practice, and competence in performing advanced clinical nursing skills. Clinical practice focuses on individuals diagnosed with psychiatric disorders and other vulnerable individuals and populations at risk with mental health disorders.

The APRN-PMH is prepared to perform all duties of the basic level psychiatric-mental health nurse. Additionally, because of educational preparation and clinical practice expertise, the APRN-PMH is able to perform complete delivery of direct primary mental health care services to clients, including, but not limited to:

- Completing a health assessment/examination.
- Conducting health screening and evaluation.
- Conducting individual, family, group, and network psychotherapy.
- Designing and conducting mental illness preventive interventions.
- Directing and providing home health services to mental health patients.
- Formulating differential diagnoses based on clinical findings.
- Formulating, implementing, and evaluating an outcome-based treatment plan.
- Planning and carrying out health promotion activities.

- Ordering, conducting, and interpreting pertinent laboratory and diagnostic studies and procedures.
- Prescribing, monitoring, managing, and evaluating psychopharmacological and related medications.
- Providing integrated mental health services in general health settings.

It is not expected that every APRN-PMH will perform all the duties listed above.

Every nurse is responsible for practicing nursing in accordance with state laws. Although a specific function is within the scope of the nurse's practice, the nurse can decide to refer a client to another clinician for that aspect of care.

### Additional Functions of the APRN-PMH

*Case management activities:* Utilization of population-specific nursing knowledge along with research, knowledge of mental health within the legal system, supportive psychotherapy expertise in obtaining necessary psychiatric care for a patient in order to maximize patient outcomes.

*Clinical supervisory responsibilities:* Providing clinical supervision, peer consultation, providing peer supervision. This is a professional and educative development process for growth. This is NOT a staff performance evaluation.

*Community interventions:* The APRN-PMH assesses the health needs of populations within the community and designs programs for at-risk populations. Attention to cultural, developmental, and environmental factors within the community is necessary.

*Consultation-liaison activities:* Consultation-liaison activities focus on emotional, developmental, spiritual, behavioral, and cognitive responses of patients in health care areas such as hospitals, rehabilitation centers, and outpatient facilities. The APRN-PMH consultation may include consultee-centered consultation—assessing and recommending actions that focus on the health care delivery organization as the client (Caplan & Caplan, 1993).

*Psychopharmacology interventions:* These interventions include prescription of pharmacological agents used to treat mental disorders and ordering and interpretation of diagnostic and laboratory tests. The APRN-PMH seeks optimal patient outcomes, anticipates side effects, and ensures against adverse drug reactions/interactions.

*Psychotherapy:* Psychotherapy is intended to alleviate emotional distress, assist in reversing or changing negative behavior, and assist in facilitating growth. Brief or long-term therapy is provided (e.g., behavioral, insight therapy, solution-focused therapy, Gestalt therapy, psychoanalytic, play therapy, and others) to individuals, couples, groups, or families.

## Standards of Care

The Standards of Care coincide with the nursing process. Please refer to ANA's *Scope and Standards of Psychiatric-Mental Health Nursing Practice* for detailed information.

### Scope of Practice for Psychiatric-Mental Health Nursing

The scope of practice for psychiatric-mental health nurses is established by the profession and published through the professional association for nurses—the American Nurses Association.

- Registered nurses are licensed and approved by their individual states to practice nursing.
- Each state has its own requirements, rules, and regulations for nursing practice.

- Some states are working towards allowing nurses the ability to work interstate to allow ease of movement.
- Certification is available at the generalist and specialist levels for psychiatric-mental health nursing.
- Additional certifications may be necessary based upon the specialization of practice (e.g., practice in marriage and family therapy, addictions counseling).

The American Nurses Association (2000) states: "Psychiatric-mental health nursing is the diagnosis and treatment of human responses to actual or potential mental health problems. Psychiatric-mental health nursing is a specialized area of nursing practice." A variety of theories assist in explaining the science of human behavior and the therapeutic use of self as the art of providing care to individuals.

Comprehensive psychiatric-mental health nursing care is delivered in a variety of settings, including:

- Intermediate and long-term care (e.g., residential care facilities, general hospitals, centers for treatment of chemical dependency and detoxification, inpatient psychiatric units, correctional facilities).* An essential role of the nurse is to assist in the client's smooth transition from the institution to the community setting.
- Community-based care (e.g., homes, schools, worksites, halfway houses, home health agencies, employee assistance programs, health maintenance organizations, senior centers, nursing homes, emergency and crisis centers, nursing homes, foster care residences, shelters and clinics for the homeless, and others).
- The delivery of health services through the technology of telecommunications removes time and distance barriers for the delivery of the health care service. The psychiatric-mental health nurse can utilize means of electronic communication, such as telephone consultation, interactive video sessions, computers, faxing, electronic mail, image transmission, research, and educational programs. The nurse needs to utilize practice approaches that are based on empirical evidence and professional consensus.

## Self-Employment

Primary mental health care is defined as "the continuous and comprehensive services necessary for promotion of optimal mental health; the prevention of mental illness; health maintenance; management of, and referral for, mental and physical health problems; the diagnosis and treatment of mental disorders and their sequelae; and rehabilitation." (Haber & Billings, 1993)

The APRN-PMH can provide direct services to clients through private practice, group practice settings, managed care companies, health provider organizations, home health agencies, and other service delivery agreements. The self-employed nurse may also provide consultation-liaison services for an organization and its staff, or may form a nurse-owned corporation or organization to compete with other providers.

---

*It is the nurse's responsibility to acquire the knowledge and skills necessary to provide the services to the subspecialty group.

The APRN-PMH is able to:

- Provide assessment.
- Diagnose, utilizing nursing diagnoses based on the North American Nursing Diagnosis Association (NANDA, 1999), the *Diagnostic and Statistical Manual of Mental Disorders of the American Psychiatric Association* (American Psychiatric Association, 2000), or the International Classification of Diseases (WHO, 1993).
- Identify outcomes.
- Plan interventions or treatment based on assessment data and theoretical hypotheses.
- Evaluate the effectiveness of the process and revise the plan of care to ensure optimal patient outcomes.

## Phenomena of Concern for Psychiatric-Mental Health Nurses

The phenomena of concern for psychiatric-mental health nurses includes actual or potential mental health problems of clients such as:

- The maintenance of optimal mental health and well-being and the prevention of mental illness.
- Self-care limitations or impaired functioning related to mental, emotional, and physiological distress.
- Deficits in the functioning of significant biological, emotional, and cognitive systems.
- Emotional stress or crisis related to illness, pain, disability, and loss.
- Self-concept and body image changes, developmental issues, life process changes, and end-of-life issues.
- Problems related to emotions such as anxiety, anger, confusion, fear, grief, loneliness, powerlessness, and sadness.
- Physical symptoms that occur along with altered physiological functioning.
- Psychological symptoms that occur along with altered physiological functioning.
- Alterations in communicating, decision-making, perceiving, symbolizing, and thinking.
- Difficulties relating to others.
- Behaviors and mental states that indicate the patient is a danger to self or others or has a severe disability.
- Symptom management, side effects/toxicities associated with self-administered drugs, psychopharmacological intervention, and other features of the treatment regimen.
- Interpersonal, environmental circumstances or events, organizational, sociocultural, and spiritual issues that have an impact on the mental and emotional well-being of the individual, family, or community.

## Subspecialization

An APRN-PMH may subspecialize in such areas as addiction, depression, serious and persistent mental illness, or may have a particular practice focus, such as community, group, couple, family, and/or individuals. The nurse may also select a specific role or function for his or her practice (e.g., case management, psychiatric consultation/liaison).

# Clinical Nurse Specialist Roles

There are six subroles that a Clinical Nurse Specialist functions within. The CNS is:
- an expert clinician
- a clinical supervisor
- an educator
- a consultant
- a researcher
- an administrator (this role will be discussed and covered in a later section).

## Advanced Clinical Practice

In the role of the expert in clinical practice, the CNS:
- Is expert and thoroughly skilled in providing care.
- Delivers care that is performed confidently and in a timely manner.
- Provides expert role modeling.
- Is aware of prevention of complications regardless of the disease process or diagnostic entity.
- Strives for personal excellence and quality patient care.
- Is an expert coach to patients.
- May or may not exercise prescriptive privileges.

*"The expert practitioner subrole must continue to be the central focus for the role of Clinical Nurse Specialist."* (Hamric & Spross, 1989)

In her theory "From Novice to Expert," Benner (1984) states that nursing practice evolves from the nurse beginning at the novice level and proceeding to the expert level of nursing practice. When an individual who has been proficient and an "expert" in providing basic level psychiatric nursing services begins to practice at the advanced level, the individual may experience a sense of frustration of starting at the "novice" level in advanced practice nursing. It is important for this individual to know that feelings of frustration occurring within the first 0–9 months are completely normal and will be alleviated as the individual feels more competent and proficient in the new role.

In the beginning, the novice CNS may only be able to focus on becoming proficient in one or two of the five subroles; however, as the nurse becomes more familiar and comfortable with that subrole, he/she will more easily "try on" and practice the other subroles.

Thirty-seven and a half percent of CNSs stated they felt they were at the novice level of practice for the first 9 months and another 37.5% of CNSs reported they were at the beginner level of practice for the first 9 months of practice. In years 1–1.9, CNSs reported being at the intermediate level of practice. At 3–4.9 years of practice as a CNS, the majority of responders felt they were at the intermediate level of practice. At 5–9.9 years as a CNS, the majority felt they were at the advanced level of practice. At 10 years, all 13 responders reported being at the advanced level of practice as a CNS (Hamric & Spross, 1989).

## Clinical Supervision

Clinical supervision is a formal process of support and learning that enables individual practitioners to develop knowledge and competence, assume responsibility for their own practice and enhance consumer protection and safety in complex situations.

## Types of Supervision

*Clinical*—enables a focus on professional competencies and increases the potential for a high standard of delivery of care to patients and their families.

*Managerial*—concerned with accountability and with the monitoring of work commissioned by an organization.

*Group*—supervision provided within a group format (e.g., professionals are accountable to one another).

*Training*—acquisition of specific skills and competencies; accountability is to the educational establishment.

For the purposes of becoming certified as a Clinical Nurse Specialist, supervision needs to be provided by someone who is regarded as having expert knowledge relevant to the focus of clinical supervision (another CNS). Another expert, for example, a psychiatrist or a psychologist, may provide some hours of supervision.

## Three Modes of Supervision

*Patient-Centered Supervision*—nurse brings to supervision problems of a technical nature.

*Clinical-centered supervision*—centers on unseen, unheard, or unspoken aspects of professional practice. The nurse is helped to reflect on events concerned with complex human dynamics and is encouraged to think about factors influencing his/her clinical practice (outside awareness).

*Process-Centered Supervision*—focuses on processes of events as they unfold between a patient, family members, or colleagues, a nurse and supervisor, and interactions between the patient and nurse (mirroring or paralleling).

### Benefits of Clinical Supervision

The concept of "Good Enough" is necessary for effective growth and development (Winnicott, 1965).

This idea refers to early experiences of beneficial mothering and a feeling of being on the inside of a relationship that is consistent (Bick, 1968).

### Other Benefits of Clinical Supervision

* Clinical supervision can influence other professional alliances, including those with patients and families (Jones, 1998);
* Clinical supervision can provide opportunities to gain valuable experiential knowledge of building and establishing constructive professional relationships;
* Clinical supervision can repair professional attitudes and restore an aptitude for work during exhausting professional demands (Yerushalmi, 1994);
* Clinical supervision can often be regarded as a means of support, personal development, and maintaining integrity;
* Clinical supervision can build confidence in the nursing role; reduce stress, burnout, and sickness levels;
* Clinical supervision can increase nurses' job satisfaction.

Benefits of clinical supervision increase with longer duration of participation in clinical supervision.

## Supervisee

- Define the guidelines within which you are to work with your supervisor in supervision.
- Discuss, explore working boundaries, confidentiality, accountability, parameters, and limits.
- Identify personal ways of gaining support more effectively, asking, for example,
  - How can I gain more support through clinical supervision and from my supervisor?
  - What do I hope to gain through clinical supervision?
  - What responsibilities do I have in clinical supervision?
  - What limits do I need/want to set in clinical supervision?
- Establish dates, times, and length of clinical supervision.
- Document exchanges.

## Effective supervisee behaviors

- Reflect on practice and implement changes as needed.
- Seek supervision and prepare by identifying cases or issues.
- Be open to change; seek input/feedback.
- Meet regularly.
- Be honest about what you do and do not know.
- Ask a lot of questions.
- Be teachable.
- Follow suggestions given in supervision.
- Listen objectively; be approachable.

## Roles of the Supervisor

- Have a close relationship with his or her own supervisor.
- Recognize when things are going well.
- Identify potential areas of difficulty.
- Devise effective ways of working with uncertainty.
- Allow time for supervisees to evaluate their practice.
- Structure the relationship and professional conversations.
- Offer a structured pathway, model, or framework for keeping the professional relationship appropriate and preventing the session from becoming "just a chat."

## Effective supervisor behaviors

- Present cases for discussion
- Co/joint interviewing
- Direct observation
- Role-play
- Audio and video recording and review
- Provide relevant literature
- Teach therapeutic skills
- Hold supervisee accountable
- Communicate directly
- Acknowledge supervisee experience/knowledge
- Be willing to listen and able to give clear direction and feedback
- Stay within the guidelines of your expertise as a supervisor
- Give honest evaluative feedback
- Encourage and affirm supervisee growth
- Discuss theoretical frameworks for approaching practice/supervision

## Establishing a Clinical Supervision Relationship

- Be aware of competing roles (e.g., manager/supervisor or boss/supervisor).
- Discuss and review individual and joint responsibilities at the beginning of the relationship.
- Negotiate and agree upon tentative working guidelines for clinical supervision.
- Take time to assess how well the process is progressing.
- Define the guidelines within which you are to work.
- Document exchanges.
- Discuss, explore working boundaries, confidentiality, accountability, parameters and limits.
- Identify personal ways of gaining support more effectively.
- Do we wish to work together?
- Can we work together?
- Do our other roles allow us to work together?
- Establish dates, times, and length of clinical supervision

## Clinical Supervision Models

The most frequently cited supervision model in nursing is by Proctor (1986). There are three supervision functions: restorative, formative, and normative.

*Restorative*—Providing support in an attempt to relieve the stress of the job of nursing
*Formative*—Educative, developing skills understanding, and ability by reflection
*Normative*—Maintenance of professional standards

Model for Clinical Supervision. Based on Heron's (1989) six-category intervention analysis framework (Chambers & Long, 1995; Fowler, 1996, and Cutcliffe & Epling, 1997).

*Other models include:*

*Prescriptive*—offer advice and make suggestions
*Informative*—offer information or instruction
*Confronting*—challenge the individual's behavior, attitudes, or beliefs
*Cathartic*—enable the release of tension and strong emotion
*Catalytic*—encourage further self-exploration, self-directed living, learning, and problem solving
*Supportive*—validate or confirm the worth and value of the client's person, qualities, attitudes, or actions.

## Cognitive Therapy Supervision Model

The principles of cognitive therapy supervision include the following:
- Aims to be focused, structured, educational, and collaborative.

- Aims to increase awareness of how our own cognitions can influence the therapeutic endeavor and how we can use our cognitions to understand the process of CT.

- Uncovers the supervisee's thoughts and feelings about his or her relationship with clients with "the added modeling effect of showing him/her how to work through similar emotions in the client."

- Acknowledges that the practice of supervisor and supervisee will be influenced by their own core beliefs, underlying assumptions, and automatic thoughts.

- Supervision sessions are structured by an agenda and aim to make links across sessions.

- Aims to summarize previous session content and review any learning that has occurred between sessions.

- May include review of audio and videotapes of supervisee's work
- Supervisor aims to help supervisees apply CT as well as they can and to develop their assessment, conceptualization, and treatment skills.

An example of a cognitive therapy supervision session agenda:
- Personal update
- Agenda setting
- Link to last supervision session
- Previously supervised cases
- Check on homework task
- Discussion of agenda items
- Assignment of new homework
- Summary and feedback from supervisee

Helpful questions for supervision (based on cognitive therapy supervision model, Sloan, White, & Coit. 2000):

| Agenda item | Possible questions for clinical supervision in Adv. PMHN |
| --- | --- |
| Personal update | How are things with you?<br>What has been happening since we last met? |
| Agenda setting | What items do you want to highlight for the agenda today?<br>How can I help you today?<br>What do you want to focus on? |
| Link to last session | What things did you find useful from our last supervision?<br>Has there been anything from our last meeting that you have incorporated into your practice? |
| Previously supervised case | Last time we talked about anxiety control for Mrs. R.<br>How is she? |
| Check on homework task | You were going to investigate some distraction techniques for anxiety control. What did you find out?<br>What have you found useful?<br>What didn't help? |
| Discussion of agenda items | Role-play the use of empathy in assessing the experience of anxiety. |
| Assignment of new homework | What strategies does the research literature suggest?<br>What have you found that works? |
| Summary and feedback from supervisee | What aspects of today's session have you found helpful/unhelpful?<br>Is there anything else I could have done to help you with this client? |

*Learning Process Supervision Model*

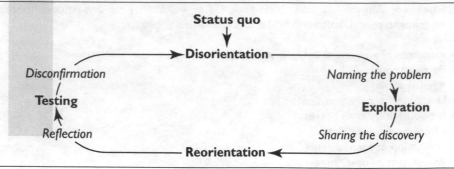

Figure 1-1. Learning process sequence (adapted from Taylor 1987).

The learner achieves a change in perspective through four stages (words in **bold**) and four phase transition points (words in *italics*).

The pivotal transition is the move from a state of equilibrium (**status quo**) to a state of **disorientation** that occurs when expectations are thwarted by experience.

The **disorientation** that follows can be intense and is usually accompanied by a crisis in confidence.

Then there is a phase during which the problem is named without blaming either oneself or others (*naming the problem*).

By *naming the problem*, the learner is liberated from the anxiety of **disorientation.**

The learner can then begin a period of **exploration,** which is "intuitively guided, collaborative and open-ended."

This process (*sharing the discovery*) enables the learner to gather insights, confidence and satisfaction."

This reflective process leads to a **reorientation**—a major insight or synthesis experience simultaneous with a new approach to the learning task.

The learner then **tests** his or her new understanding by sharing the discovery with others.

A stage of **equilibrium** then follows "in which the new perspective and approach is elaborated, refined and applied." (Taylor, 1987)

## Additional Comments Regarding Clinical Supervision

- Clinical supervision and therapy are generally considered to be in opposition.
- When the nurse benefits from the learning experiences that occur within clinical supervision, it can be considered therapeutic.
- Professional and personal self cannot be separated (Heath & Freshwater, 2000).
- If the supervision relationship is supportive and helpful, positive changes can occur in self-confidence, self-perception, and self-affirmation.

## Education

Within the subrole of educator, the CNS:
- Teaches individuals, couples, families, systems, and communities.
- Teaches within schools of nursing, colleges.
- Provides information to resolve health problems and improve the quality of care.
- Functions as a role model and preceptor for nurse generalists and for faculty and students in a variety of clinical arenas:
  - provides input and critique for curriculum development;
  - teaches specific content in nursing programs—preceptor, resource person, program planner, and lecturer in education of undergraduate and graduate students;
  - teaches in continuing education programs (e.g., written programs and/or inservices provided for continuing education units (CEUs) or community education programs); and
  - teaches in other disciplines (e.g., medicine, social work).
- Follows adult learning principles.

## Adult Learning Theory

In the teaching and learning process,
- Teaching = creating an environment where learning can occur.
- The teacher is the facilitator.
- The teacher needs to guide the learning.
- Learning = change.
- The learner has the responsibility to do the learning.
- Learning is active, experiential, and holistic, involving the individual and his or her environment.
- Teaching is the facilitation of learning, which involves a sharing and mutual experience of learning on the part of both teacher and learner.

## Teaching Strategies

- Select a topic of acute interest—individuals rarely forget a presentation by an impassioned teacher.
- Establish clear and measurable goals and objectives for the presentation. Ask yourself, "What do I hope the learner(s) will take from the presentation?" Setting presentation goals and objectives will guide you in planning content, plus it will save preparation time. (A general rule of thumb is that for each 50 minutes of presentation, plan 4 hours for preparation of the material.)
- Complete a literature search and get necessary materials together before developing the content. This will save you time in the long run.
- Organize the material in a systematic fashion—ordering of information increases the ease with which learning takes place.
- Know your audience and gear the presentation to the members of the audience.
- Select appropriate teaching strategies (e.g., lecture and discussion, case study presentations, role-play, role modeling, seminars, speaker panel, use of relevant examples from clinical practice, gaming/simulation, peer discussions).
- Use a variety of teaching aids. They greatly enhance and complement a presentation and will keep learners actively engaged (e.g., slides, handouts, etc.).

If possible, assess learner needs at the beginning of or prior to the presentation.

## Domains of Learning
- Cognitive learner
- Kinesthetic learner = learns by doing (provide experiential exercises, e.g., role-playing)
- Affective learner = learns by feeling
- Visual learner = learns by seeing
- Auditory learner = learns by hearing

Neurolinguistic Programming (NLP) provides several verbal and nonverbal approaches to determine if an individual learns better through use of visual, auditory, or kinesthetic (sensory) means.

Please keep these concepts in mind when you are planning teaching interventions for your client(s) or student(s):

*Visual learner*—The learner may say, "That looks good to me," or "I see what you mean." The visual learner may also look up to the ceiling as if looking for the answers (visual processing).

*Auditory learner*—The learner may say, "That sounds like an interesting topic," or "I hear what you are saying." The auditory learner may also look towards the side as if listening for the answer (auditory processing).

*Kinesthetic (sensory) learner*—The learner may say, "I sense that this is a touchy subject for you"; other senses may be implied, such as: "That stinks," "I feel this is not a good time," "That leaves a bad taste in my mouth."

Once you have assessed the type of learner with whom you are working, you can then use the same language that the learner is using. When learners hear you use their language, they are more apt to think: "He/she really understands me. He/she seems a lot like me."

## Evaluation
Types of evaluation include:
- Formative evaluation: written words placed on an evaluation.
- Summative evaluation: essential points, adding all key points from individual evaluations and compiling them into one evaluation.

For example: After providing a presentation on "Assessing, Diagnosing and Interventions in the Care of Depressed Older Adults," the sponsor of the program had participants fill out a formative evaluation of the program. The sponsor then compiled the evaluations and provided the presenter with the results in a written format (summative evaluation).

### Things to Remember
- Objectives must be measurable and attainable.
- Documentation is important.
- Changes occur in the learner as a result of aging.

## The Learning Process

Learning is:

- An active and continuous process, manifested by growth and changes in behavior.
- Dependent upon the readiness, emotional state, abilities, and potential of the learner.
- Influenced by the life experiences of the learner.
- Facilitated when information to be learned has relevance to the learner.
- Facilitated by proceeding from the simple to the complex and from the known to the unknown.
- Facilitated when the learner can test ideas, analyze mistakes, take risks, and be creative.
- Enabling the student to deal with the expansion of knowledge and changes in nursing and society.
- Facilitated when the learner has knowledge of his/her progress toward the goal.
- Enhanced in situations in which satisfaction is derived.
- Determined by the kind of social, emotional, and intellectual behavior that emerges from the learning situation.
- Facilitated by recognition of similarities and differences between past experiences and present situations.
- Influenced by the learner's perception of self and the situation in which he/she finds himself/herself.
- More effective when there is immediate application of what is being taught.
- Helped by determining what kind of learning experiences will be most effective in terms of time and effort.
- Most effective when self-directed and when it applies to the learner's daily activities.
- Most effective when the learner is motivated to learn.
- Best accomplished when individuals are allowed to pursue their own areas of interest at their own rate and to find answers to questions on their own.
- A continuous process, improved by doing.
- Reinforced when appealing to several senses. Individuals remember:
  - 10% of what they read
  - 20% of what they hear
  - 30% of what they see
  - 50% of what they see and hear
  - 80% of what they say
  - 90% of what they say while doing

## Consultation

The CNS is the consultant. The consultee is the one who has identified a problem and who recognizes that the consultant has specialized expertise to apply to the problem and initiates the consultation. Usually consultation is sought for advice about a patient-related problem. An example would be a nursing home (consultee) that has identified it has many patients who have behavioral problems. The home calls a CNS (consultant) to assist in solving the problem. Consultation is an interactive, supportive, interpersonal process in which the consultant collaborates with the consultee who has requested assistance with problem solving. The consultant typically has NO direct authority or evaluative responsibilities over the consultee.

The consultant's authority is based on "expert knowledge." The consultation process is NOT psychotherapy, but it can be therapeutic. The CNS consultant follows the nursing process to assist in collecting data, developing a nursing diagnosis, and providing recommendations/interventions.

Skills and knowledge needed by the CNS consultant include:
• Consultation process (follow the nursing process)
• Systems theory
• Communications
• Change theory
• Nursing Process
• Problem solving
• Conflict resolution
• Adult learning theory
• Group process

Consultation facilitates an interdisciplinary approach to client care and assists in problem solving with individual emotional and/or situational crises, families, groups, agencies, communities, and colleagues. Consultation identifies problem etiologies, such as:
• Provider competence
• Facility
• Equipment
• Service delivery systems

## Internal Consultant/External Consultant

*Internal Consultant*
The CNS evaluates a medical patient secondary to a psychiatric problem (e.g., in a hospital setting, a patient is admitted for delirium. A CNS may be consulted to make recommendations about possible psychiatric causes, ideas for lab tests to be completed and considered, and recommendations for care).

The CNS is called upon for a professional opinion related to staffing issues (e.g., morale, group process, direction on ethical and legal issues).

*External Consultant*
The CNS may provide advice regarding appropriateness of potential referrals for psychiatric home care.

The CNS may provide clinical suggestions for managing difficult behaviors in the home setting/nursing home.

The CNS may be an organizational consultant. The CNS collects data related to the problem from employees and administration. Based on the data collected, the CNS makes a nursing diagnosis, suggests interventions for improvement, and provides evaluation criteria. (One CNS I know provided consultation to an organization and found that the CEO had symptoms of clinical depression. The CEO was referred for psychiatric evaluation and treatment and it assisted in resolving the problem for which the CNS was consulted.)

## Interdisciplinary/Intradisciplinary Consultation

*Interdisciplinary Consultation*
- Accept different perspectives within the organization in which you are consulting.
- Be able to function interdependently.
- Remember, roles are negotiated between team members.
- Constantly review and challenge ideas.
- Take risks.
- Possess personal identity and integrity.
- Accept the team's philosophy of care.
- Establish new interaction patterns.
- Accept changes in authority and status.
- Develop methods of conflict resolution and decision making.

*Intradisciplinary Consultation*
- A peer or colleague relationship in which the consultee, NOT the consultant, defines the problem.
- Usually brief, a short series of visits.
- Increases the capacity of the consultee to master future, similar problems.
- The consultant does not counsel staff but refers for counseling if that is the problem.
- Remember, the consultee does not have to take your advice.

## Collaboration

Collaboration includes developing relationships with key individuals and developing collaborative relationships with individuals who know key individuals. Collaboration strategies include:

- Planning inservices.
- Coaching individual staff members to develop assertiveness and conflict resolution skills.
- Developing and participating in specific programs requiring collaboration.
- Making oneself indispensable to the parties involved (work effectively with patients whom other caregivers find difficult to manage).
- Developing scope of practice statements for institutions that employ CNSs.
- Developing clinical protocols in joint practice committees.
- Being instrumental in identifying situations that would benefit from standing clinical protocols.
- Engaging in joint review of medical records.

## Consultation Process—Conceptualized in Terms of the Nursing Process

The four phases of consultation are:
- Entry, beginning of the consultation request.
- Diagnosis.
- Response or intervention.
- Closure and evaluation.

Steps of consultation as outlined by Caplan, 1970:
- Assessment of the consultation problem following the consultation request (similar to assessment in the nursing process).

* The consultation report (similar to providing the nursing diagnosis and interventions for implementation).
* Implementation of the consultant's request.
* Follow-up (similar to evaluation in the nursing process).

*Types of Mental Health Consultation*
* *Client-centered—assists in improving the consultee's knowledge and skills to enhance his or her handling of similar problems in the future.
* *Consultee-centered
* Program-centered administrative
* Consultee-centered administrative

*Most readily employed by the psychiatric consultant-liaison nurse.

Goals of consultation/liaison activities are complementary and interdependent. Consultation and liaison activities are inseparable areas of clinical practice. Within the liaison process, there is a linkage of health care professionals to facilitate communication between clients, families, and specific health care professionals.

Examples of consultation/liaison activities include:
* Unit-based education programs (teaching nurses about alcohol and drug withdrawal and treatment).
* Patient education programs (teaching patients about assertiveness, Seasonal Affective Depression).
* Participation in discharge planning.
* Nursing care planning.
* Facilitation of patient, family, or staff nurse support groups (assisting in starting a lupus support group within the community).

Characteristics helpful in psychiatric consultant-liaison nursing:
* Acceptance of ambiguous situations.
* Tolerance of personal rejections.
* Capacity and willingness to tolerate consistently stressful and often unpredictable, difficult situations with clients, families, and healthcare providers.

## The CNS as a Change Agent

The CNS is a facilitator of change. The definition of "change" is "to make different or modify." A change agent is one who works to make, modify, or make something different than the status quo.

Facilitators of change include:
* A desire to change
* Motivation to change
* Positive past experience with change
* Not perceiving change as a threat
* Trust in the change agent
* A change that can be clearly communicated and described
* Support and involvement from others
* Adequate resources

- An accurate diagnosis of the problem
- A solution appropriate to the problem
- Determining what roles will be assumed

Planned change is a conscious, deliberate, and collaborative effort to improve the operations of a human system, whether it be a self, social, or cultural system, through utilization of valid knowledge (Bennis, 1976).

Change strategies include power/coercive, normative/re-educative, and empirical/rational. The consultant should:

- Choose a strategy depending on the anticipated maturity (competence and motivation) of followers.
- Foster independence by maximizing strengths.
- Determine desired level of functioning.
- Have realistic expectations.

The change agent should also realize:
- Independence is a long process.
- Acute patients need nurturing; less nurturing is needed with higher functioning patients.
- Behavior that has been useful over long periods of time takes time to change.
- Change will be resisted and at times may be sabotaged.
- Coping skills need to be adequate to deal with growth.
- Realistic goals depend on other supports in the community.
- The family should be involved.

## Satir and Change

There is no need to focus on the extinction of old learning because change will occur through the additive process of transformation and atrophy. By focusing on a new way of doing things or of coping that is better than the old way, the individual will start using the new way and the old way will die of disuse.

The process of learning is enhanced and maximized when the individual feels supported and thus willing and able to take risks.

When individuals are exposed to new behavioral learning, they need to take for themselves only that which fits for them, rejecting knowledge with which they are not comfortable (similar to 12-step support groups that say, "Take what you like and leave the rest.")

Satir believes the learning process is essentially a discovery or, more accurately, a rediscovery by the learner of knowledge that is already within, and that the answers to questions are found within the individual who asks them. The role of the therapist is to use strategic questions to help the client find his/her own answers.

Barriers to change:
- A desire to maintain the status quo
- Satisfaction with the status quo
- Change is perceived as a threat
- Lack of motivation to change
- Negative past experience with change
- Lack of trust in the change agent

- Poor communication
- Change is of an abstract nature so difficult to communicate clearly
- Lack of support from others
- Inadequate resources
- Unrealistic, incongruent solution
- Fear of failure
- A lack of understanding as to what is needed to change

The Johari window (Luft, 1984) (below) is an awareness model that can assist the CNS in understanding the principles of change. Within this model, consciousness refers to what is felt within oneself. Awareness refers to what is felt outside oneself.

Table 1-3. Johari Window

|  | Known to self | Not known to self |
| --- | --- | --- |
| Known to others | Quadrant 1<br>Open | Quadrant 2<br>Blind |
| Not known to others | Quadrant 3<br>Hidden | Quadrant 3<br>Unknown |

Quadrant 1 is the open quadrant, which refers to behavior, feelings, and motivation that is known to self and to others.

Quadrant 2 is the blind quadrant, which refers to behavior, feelings, and motivation that is known to others but not to self.

Quadrant 3 is the hidden quadrant, which refers to behavior, feelings and motivation that is known to self, but not to others.

Quadrant 4 is the unknown quadrant, which refers to behavior, feelings and motivation that is unknown to self and others.

Principles of change utilizing the Johari window (Luft, 1984) include:
- A change in one quadrant will affect all other quadrants. (e.g., if a patient begins to share hidden thoughts and feelings with a therapist, quadrant 3 becomes smaller and the patient becomes more open and quadrant 1 becomes larger).
- It takes energy to deny, hide, stifle, or be blind to one's personal behavior and its effect on relationships.
- Mutual trust tends to increase awareness. Threats from others tend to decrease personal awareness. If a therapist comes across to the client as threatening, the client will not be as open to self-disclosing and will be less open to reveal hidden material/issues.
- Forced awareness or exposure to issues or behavior is undesirable and is mostly ineffective (e.g., forcing or demanding that a client look at the issue of alcohol dependence will only cause the alcoholic client to continue to deny the behavior).

- When interpersonal learning occurs, it means that a change has taken place. Quadrant 1 becomes larger (the client becomes more open) and one or more of the other quadrants become smaller.
- The smaller the first quadrant, the poorer the communication. A client with a small first quadrant, or lack of openness, will spend a lot of time and energy in one or more of the other quadrants. A client with narcissistic personality disorder, for example, will spend a lot of energy in quadrant 3 by hiding feelings of insecurity and projecting a "better than all others" attitude. The client is less open with disclosing thoughts and feelings and individuals may find it difficult to relate to him or her.
- Respect and be sensitive to the desire of others to keep quadrant 2 (blind to self), quadrant 3 (hidden to others), and quadrant 4 (unknown to self and others).

*Planned Changed Process*
- Assess situation
- Collect data
- Analyze data
- Plan change strategy
- Implement change
- Evaluate effectiveness
- Stabilize change

## Demonstrating Creativity as a CNS
- Creativity involves looking at familiar things/situations and thinking or seeing something different or unique.

*Why don't individuals think creatively or differently more often?*
- Creativity is not required in jobs, organizations, friends, and colleagues.
- Predictability and rationality are valued in society.
- Time, space, energy, and resources do not allow individuals to get in a creative mind-set.
- Mental locks keep individuals from having creative ideas.

*More Thoughts on Creativity*
- Creativity is about the quality of originality that leads to new ways of seeing things/ideas.
- Creativity is the thinking process associated with imagination, insight, invention, innovation, ingenuity, intuition, inspiration and illumination.
- The related term to creativity is innovation.
- As a CHANGE AGENT, encourage innovation.
- Ask, "Why do we do it this way?"
- Consciously search for opportunities to innovate.
- Set up meetings and other forms of communications for sharing and discussing ideas.
- Introduce techniques such as brainstorming to stimulate ideas.
- Set up incentive schemes to encourage new ideas.
- Send staff to conferences where new ideas are being discussed.

## Research
Definition:
* Nursing research is concerned with finding a body of knowledge and practice that is unique to nursing.
* A theoretical framework within which to intelligently base practice.
* A true profession pushes back its own frontiers to greater knowledge and conducts its own investigations to enhance social and personal well-being of individuals.

### Goals of Nursing Research
* Promote scientific inquiry in clinical practice
* Use research findings to improve practice.
* Contribute to research in their specialization by:
  * generating and refining research questions,
  * interpreting research findings and applying them to clinical practice,
  * educating other nurses about research findings,
  * collaborating with nurse researchers, nurse educators, and nurse theorists, and
  * communicating research findings through publication.

### Purpose and Values of Nursing Research
* To describe a state of affairs
* To explore problem areas
* To determine solutions for problems
* To predict cause and effect and/or co-relationships

### Formulating a Research Question
* Consider ethical implications
* Consider access to subjects
* Consider cost (equipment, supplies, time, etc.)
* Consider cooperation of others that will be needed
* Consider your own experience
* Identify what you have a passion about in nursing practice

### Review of Related Literature
* Conceptual framework
* Theoretical framework

### Clarify the Purpose of the Study
A hypothesis needs to be present only in scientific research studies. It is a statement of the researcher's expected outcome based on his/her rationale. Hypotheses are not proven, only tested. Normally in a hypothesis there are dependent and independent variables.

*Independent Variable:* The independent variable is considered the cause, and it occurs first. It is a stimulus or activity that is used to create an effect on the dependent variable.

*Dependent Variable:* The dependent variable depends on and occurs after the independent variable. The dependent variable is affected by the independent variable. It is the variable of interest, the one you want to explain or predict.

*Table 1-4. Examples of Independent and Dependent Variables*

*Example #1:* Elders who participate in the decision for institutional placement are less likely to experience weight loss immediately after institutional placement than are elders who do not participate in the decision

Independent variable = participation in the decision for institutional placement
Dependent variable = the experience of weight loss

*Example #2:* Elders who experience a weight loss immediately after institutional placement are less likely to have participated in the decision for institutional placement than are elders who do not experience a weight loss.

Independent variable = the experience of weight loss
Dependent variable = participation in the decision-making process for institutional placement.

Operational definition:
Examples:
• Elder - how old?
• weight loss - how much?

The design is the plan or organization of the study, the "blueprint" to maximize the control of the study. Plan elements may include:
• Manipulation
• Randomization—assignment of subjects to groups
• Control conditions:
  • Constancy of conditions
  • Manipulation of the independent variable
  • Comparison group
  • Randomization
  • Extraneous individual characteristics

Study population for research:
• The target population must be delineated: individuals or things that meet the designated set of criteria of interest to the investigator.
• The sample population represents a miniature of the larger population. This is the group that is usually available to use in a study, and who meet the criteria of the target population.
• Probability sampling: The investigator can specify for each element of the population the probability that it will be included in the sample. Sampling units are selected by chance, and neither the investigator nor the population elements have any conscious influence on what is the final sample. (Simple random sampling, stratified random sampling, or cluster sampling are considered in this category.)
• Nonprobability sampling: The investigator has no ability to estimate the probability that each element of population can or will be a part of the sample—or even that it has a chance of being included. Nonprobability samples do not permit generalization

beyond the current study group. Confounding factors may influence this type of sampling more than random sampling, making the findings of less potential value to a broader population.

- Convenience sampling or "accident sampling" is simply taking those individuals who are available—they are in the right place at the right time.

- In purposive sampling or "judgment sampling" the investigator establishes certain criteria and subjects are selected according to these criteria.

- Quota sampling is similar to convenience sampling, but with some controls to prevent overloading with subjects having certain characteristics (it allows only a certain number or percentage of any given characteristic group).

## Sample Size Considerations

- Target population size.
- It is desirable for generalization to occur beyond the study population group.
- Outcomes for decision-making are important.
- Rule of thumb! Use a large enough sample to be representative of your target population group.
- Use the largest group you can within the constraints you have determined for the study.
- The larger the sample, the less error in measurement, the more significant and generalizable the findings.
- If using a homogeneous group (similar in characteristics), the smaller the sample size may be.
- An N (number) of less than 35–40 subjects reduces ability to use strong, powerful statistical treatment of the data.

## Informed Consent

Protection of Human Subjects in Biomedical and Behavioral Research was established by Congress in 1974. The law requires a true informed consent by any individual before becoming a subject in a research project. The informed consent must provide knowledge about:

- the nature and purpose of the research study;
- the duration of the research study;
- the methods and procedures by which the data will be collected;
- how the data will be used;
- all inconveniences, potential harm, or discomfort that might reasonably be expected from the study;
- the result, effects, and side effects that may result from participation in the study;
- the right to stop participation in the study at any time; and
- the expectation that data will remain confidential.

## Characteristics of Research (for data gathering)

Three important attributes of data gathering instruments are validity, reliability, and usability.

*Validity* is how well a test or instrument measures what it is supposed to measure. It evaluates what it is supposed to evaluate. It is a true measure of something (some variable/ characteristic); for example, a test may be reliable (measure consistently) without being valid BUT a valid test may not be considered valid unless it has both reliability and validity—it must measure consistently what it is supposed to measure. **Validity is the most important characteristic of a measuring device.** Validity is never 100%. Something always falls short in some way or another. It is important to determine whether the validity of an instrument is sufficient to be used for the purpose of the particular study under investigation.

*Reliability* means how well a measuring instrument measures something—it means how consistent it is in measuring something. Reliability is usually expressed as a coefficient number: 1.00–100% reliable. Most instruments are less than perfect. A correlation coefficient of 0.80 or higher is considered an acceptable level of reliability for a measure. The amount of reliability needed is determined by the purpose for which the instrument is used and the vital/crucial decision that will be made from the findings. The more crucial the decision-making, the more validity and reliability are needed to have confidence in the measure. A less than perfect validity or reliability are due to errors in measurement. These include conditions affecting the test situation, the subject taking the instrument, and the problems with the instrument itself.

An instrument may be reliable (able to measure something consistently) without being valid (appropriate instrument for the measures desired). Validity requires that an instrument be also reliable to be valid.

Research is only as good as the research-gathering instruments used on an appropriate population group/sample. No matter how well the research question/problem is delineated or hypotheses generated, the outcomes of a study depend upon the appropriateness of measures used, their validity and reliability, and the extent to which effective, useful data analysis techniques can make the findings meaningful and useful for predetermined purposes.

PRETESTING self-developed instruments is a must! Pretesting on a population sample similar to the one planned for the study is essential. Evaluating the strengths and weaknesses of an instrument with adequate revisions assures proper use of data-gathering instruments.

## Data Gathering

Data (information) must be obtained in any type of study to answer the question(s) and or problem(s) under investigation. Data may be of two types:

- Qualitative: Words—descriptions in narrative form, concepts, facts, verbatim statements of the subjects; linguistic approaches.
- Quantitative: Numbers—quantification enhances precision of studies.

  Comparisons with quantitative data are much less subjective and much of the time qualitative data can be converted to numerical categories. This in essence usually takes ordinal data (orders, ranks, etc.) of narrative differences and changes them. Numbers are much easier to work with than words. Statistical analysis techniques can be used with numbers, but seldom with words/narrative data.

The need for precision and potential for any type of data to be exact and in small continuous units lends greater measurement potential and power to any statistical treatment of data. However, in nursing research, some areas of frequent study are concerned with of "wellness," "illness," and other variables not easily amenable to quantification.

## Levels of Measurement

*Nominal*—numbers can be given to names
*Ordinal*—numbers are given to rank (e.g., self-esteem on a scale from 1–10)
*Interval*—numbers have meaning as numbers
*Ratio*—numbers can be analyzed.

## Why nurses should be able to use research and statistical methods

- To read literature and studies with scrutiny and skill to apply findings in their clinical practice and work environments.
- To conduct research in nursing to take the science of nursing back to basic scientific foundations and to make new applied research applications to patient needs.
- To move nursing from intuitive, artistic ways of knowing to replicable and tested ways of deliberate nursing interventions in patient care.
- To move nursing closer to other applied health fields in basic foundations and tested practices.
- To collaborate with colleagues in medicine, etc., to seek better healthcare practices for humanity.

## Types of Research

- Basic: experimental, rolls back knowledge on "what is" in a discipline (fundamental science, etc).
- Applied: applies practical aspects of basic research findings, not purely theoretical.

## Research Outcomes

Scientific research leads to findings that can be generalized, leading to new theories, concepts, and principles. The different types of research and their goals are listed below, along with definitions of reporting mechanisms.

*Demonstration Research*—seeks to prove to others that facts already accepted really exist (already have the answer to the problem; it doesn't test hypotheses as in real, scientific research). Hunches are not operationalized.

*Replication Research*—sets out to repeat or reproduce a research project to see if the findings are correct, the same in the same or in a different setting. Tries to do again what was once done to determine reliability of findings from the first study.

*Evaluation Research*—an analysis of a program, project, agency in terms of specific goals or objectives and results of something to see if things were accomplished as the program stated it was to be done (e.g., Joint Commission on Accreditation of Healthcare Organizations [JCAHO]; NLN accreditation).

## Mean, Median, Mode

Measures of central tendency. The purpose is to isolate one response that is representative of the sample:

- To arrive at the mean, total the scores of the sample, then divide the total by the number of scores in the sample. It represents the average score of the sample. This measurement is used with interval or ratio data.
- The median is simply a point on a scale, with half of the total scores above the point and half of the scores below the point. This measurement is used with ordinal data or any rating scale.
- The mode indicates the category that occurs with greatest frequency. This measurement is the only appropriate measurement for nominal data.

## Standard Deviation

Standard deviation measures the distance of each subject from the group mean. Like the mean, this measure requires interval or ratio data. Measures of variation describe how widely individuals in a sample vary. Standard deviation is the sum of the variations of all members in a class (group) from the class mean, an average of the average (a measure of variance in a group of data). It reveals how students differ from each other in terms of the class average on a test. It is useful in assigning grades.

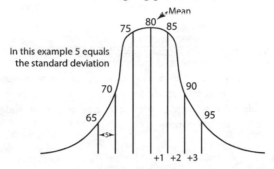

This demonstrates that 95 is 3 standard deviations from the mean (80).

## Inferential Statistics

In explanatory studies, it is not enough to just describe the data. Conclusions must be drawn from the data. Statistical inference is the process of generalizing, from sample observation, the probability of it applying to a whole population.

The overall aim of explanatory research is to determine the acceptability of the hypotheses.

## Criteria Checklist for a Research Study
• The title is readily understood
• The title is clear
• The title is clearly related to content

## The research problem
• is introduced early in the proposal
• questions to be answered are stated precisely
• the problem statement is clear
• hypotheses are stated in a form that permits them to be tested
• limitations of the study can be identified
• assumptions of the study can be identified
• pertinent terms are/can be operationally defined
• significance of the problem is discussed
• research is justified

## Review of the Literature
• cited literature is pertinent to the research problem
• relationship of the problem to previous research is made clear
• a conceptual framework/theoretical rationale is clearly stated

## Methodology

*Subjects*
- subject population (sampling frame) is described
- sampling method is described
- sampling method is justified (especially for nonprobability sampling)
- sampling size is sufficient
- standards for protection of subjects are discussed

*Instruments*
- relevant reliability data from previous research are presented
- reliability data pertinent to presented study are reported
- relevant previous validity data from previous research are presented
- validity data pertinent to present study are reported
- methods of data collection are sufficiently described to permit judgment of their appropriateness to the present study

*Design*
- design is appropriate to study questions and/or hypotheses
- proper controls are included where appropriate
- variables are/can be identified
- description of design is explicit enough to permit replication

*Data Collection*
- information presented is sufficient to answer research questions
- statistical tests to be used are identified.

# Nursing Theories

## Peplau's Theory

Hildegard Peplau wrote one of the first systematic frameworks for psychiatric nursing and focused on the nurse-client relationship. Her theory draws from developmental, interpersonal, and learning theories. She defines nursing as: "a significant, therapeutic, interpersonal process that aims to promote a patient's health in the direction of creative, constructive, productive, personal, and community living." She describes several phases of the nurse-client relationship. The phases are overlapping and the nurse and patient have changing goals and roles as the relationship progresses. The phases of the relationship that she describes are: orientation, identification, exploitation, and resolution (Peplau, 1952).

## Orem's Self-Care Model

Dorothea Orem developed a theory that nursing is based upon the patient's or the community's self-care deficit. Nurses provide assistance to individuals and systems which, because of health conditions, cannot provide self-care. Self-care deficits occur when health-related problems require nursing care (Orem, 1980).

## Johnson's Systems Model

Dorothy Johnson constructed a theoretical model on the premise that man is a behavioral system comprised of eight subsystems of behavior. General systems theory, which is discussed elsewhere, applies and overlaps with this theory. There are several major concepts in Johnson's model. Individuals are bio-psycho-socio-cultural beings. They strive continually to maintain behavioral system balance. This balance is called homeostasis. Individuals seek to maintain balance with some degree of regularity and consistency of behavior. They also actively seek new experiences, which may disturb their behavioral system balance temporarily. Johnson's perspective is that the individual is an open system with eight broadly defined subsystems, interacting with the environment by receiving input and displaying behavioral output. Disruptions in one subsystem may cause disruption in one or several other subsystems. All subsystems need to be assessed for possible changes in system stability (Johnson, 1980).

The eight subsystems identified by Johnson are:
• Ingestive: Taking in nourishment in socially and culturally acceptable ways
• Eliminative: Ridding system of waste in socially and culturally acceptable ways.
• Dependence: Self-dependence and interdependence.
• Affiliative: Security.
• Achievement: Mastery of self and environment according to an internalized standard of excellence.
• Aggressive-Protective: Survival.
• Sexual-Reproductive: Procreation and gratification.
• Restorative: Rest and sleep.

## Therapeutic Relationships

*Therapeutic Communication*
Effective communication is essential for any interaction between a nurse and a patient. In the field of psychiatric nursing, this moves to an even deeper level and the communication and interactions can be the therapy. It is important to be able to keep in mind techniques that are therapeutic and effective and those that are less so. The following is a review of some therapeutic communication techniques and some blocks to therapeutic communication.

*Therapeutic Communication Techniques*
*Broad Opening Statements*—Broad, open-ended statements such as: "If there is something bothering you I would be happy to listen," allows the patient to set the direction of the conversation.

*General Leads*—"Yes." "Oh." "Go on." Acknowledge that you are listening and understand what the patient is saying. These leads encourage the patient to keep talking. Don't overuse these, however or patient may feel interrupted or rushed.

*Reflecting*—This is the technique of repeating all or part of what the patient has said. This encourages the patient to continue and helps to clarify that what you heard is what was said. For example, if the patient says: "Everyone here hates me," the nurse might say: "Everyone here hates you?"

*Selective Reflecting*—In selective reflecting the nurse takes a more directive approach to guiding the conversation. Select the most important idea contained in what the patient has said and direct it back to the patient. For example, if the patient says: "I feel tired, I don't like it here," the nurse might respond: "Tired?" to explore the first part of the statement or: "You don't like it here?" to explore the second part.

*Clarifying*—The nurse immediately asks for clarification if any part of what the patient has said has not been understood to prevent misunderstandings.

*Sharing Observations*—Nurses share their observations regarding the patient's behavior as a way to help the patient understand his or her emotions. For example: "Your hands are shaking." "You seem upset."

*Acknowledging the Patient's Feelings*—This indicates that the patient's feelings are understood and accepted. This also encourages patients to continue expressing their emotions.

*Using Silence*—This is remaining silent and attentive. Out of this silence often emerge the feelings that the patient is dealing with. Sometimes the nurse's own discomfort can make it difficult to allow the silence.

*Giving Information*—As nurses we educate and provide specific information. Studies have shown that a major cause of anxiety in hospitalized patients is lack of information or misconceptions about their condition, treatment, or hospital routine. Education is a primary nursing function.

*Verbalizing Implied Thoughts and Feelings*—The nurse voices what the patient seems to have implied. An example: Patient: "It's a waste of time doing these exercises." Nurse: "You feel that they aren't benefiting you?"

*Validating*—Don't assume the patient's needs have been met by your intervention. Ask the patient: "Are you getting what you need or want?"

### Blocks to Therapeutic Communication and Alternatives
*Using Reassuring Clichés*—Such statements as: "You're doing just fine" minimize the patient's concerns. Don't offer false reassurance. Share your observations instead and let the patient interpret.

*Giving Advice*—Direct advice imposes the nurse's own opinions and solutions on the patient and is inappropriate. Clarify and use other communication techniques to help patients come to their own solutions.

*Giving Approval or Agreeing with the Patient*—This can be a useful response or can be a block to communication by changing the focus of the discussion to the nurse's values or feelings. Try silence or reflection.

*Requesting an Explanation*—By requesting an explanation, the nurse asks the patient to immediately analyze and explain his or her feelings or actions. Patients can't always do this. Stay with the feelings instead. It takes time for patients to come to their conclusions and interpretations. Don't rush the process.

*Expressing Disapproval*—This imposes the nurse's values onto the patient and implies that the nurse is entitled to make a negative value judgment regarding the patient's feelings or behavior. Express your input as giving information, then share your personal reactions with a colleague or friend.

*Minimizing or Belittling the Patient's Feeling*—Statements such as: "I know just how you feel" or "Everyone gets depressed sometimes" deny the importance of the patient's feelings as unique. Each individual reacts and responds differently. This approach also shifts the focus from the patient to the nurse (I know ... ) or others (Everyone gets ... ). Use acknowledging the patient's feelings or sharing information instead.

*Disagreeing with the Patient*—"You're wrong." "That's not true." Although this can by used appropriately as a reality check, it can indicate that what the patient said has not been accepted. Use giving information techniques instead.

*Stereotyped Comment*—Trite sayings such as: "How are you today?" or "Isn't it a beautiful day?" keep the conversation at a superficial level. This may be appropriate in the beginning until rapport is established. Try starting with a broad opening statement instead. Patients are in your care for a reason, not to be socially superficial.

*Changing the Subject*—The nurse directs the course of the conversation. This may make the patient feel unimportant and abandoned. Sometimes it occurs when the nurse is uncomfortable with the topic. Identify the source of your discomfort and work it through—then you will be able to use silence and really listen.

## Defense Mechanisms and Coping Strategies

All individuals must deal with the difficulties presented in life. We need ways to adjust and adapt to conflicts and stresses. Defenses mechanisms serve several purposes. They are used to make us "look better" to others, to help us to be loved and accepted. They are also used to achieve success and recognition. Mostly they help us handle tensions and anxieties.

Psychological literature defines ways that individuals defend against the unwanted and cope with events. Individuals tend to develop patterns of defense and coping, some healthy and some unhealthy. A process in therapy is to help the patient identify his or her defense mechanisms and coping strategies and if they are working and healthy or not. The patient can then broaden his or her repertoire and try new, different, more effective, and healthier ways to cope and defend.

*Coping strategies* are external responses to a stressful situation. They are problem solving. *Defense mechanisms* are an internal and often unconscious process.

### Defense Mechanisms

*Rationalization*—This is the process whereby one expresses the reason for a behavior to justify it.

*Suppression*—The conscious dismissal of an unacceptable idea, desire, painful memory, etc. from the mind.

*Denial*—The refusal to acknowledge.

*Repression*—An unconscious process that prevents or hinders an idea, desire, memory, etc. from reaching consciousness.

*Regression*—A return to an earlier stage of development.

*Fantasy*—Use of playful imagination.

*Projection*—Unconscious attribution to another of one's own thoughts, feelings, or actions.

*Dissociation*—To keep something separate and apart in one's mind.

*Conversion*—Changing of one thing into another, e.g., emotional pain becomes a physical manifestation.

*Displacement*—Transference of emotion from the original idea it was associated with to a different idea.

*Introjection*—Identification of the self with another or with some object, thereby assuming the supposed feelings of the other individual.

### Coping Strategies

*Isolation*—Placing oneself apart and alone.

*Splitting*—The process of pitting one individual against another to avoid focus on oneself.

*Devaluing*—Minimizing the individual attempting to help or intervene to avoid the issue.

*Substitution*—Turning from an obstructed or inappropriate desire to one whose gratification is socially acceptable.

*Sublimation*—Conversion of unwanted aggressive or sexual drives into socially acceptable channels.

*Compensation*—Seeking a substitute for something lacking or unacceptable.

*Over-Compensation*—The process by which a individual substitutes an opposite trait or exerts efforts in excess of that needed to compensate.

*Identification*—To consider as being the same or as being necessarily associated.

*Symbolism*—Everything that occurs is interpreted as a symbol of the patient's own thoughts.

# Legal Aspects of Care

### Patient Rights

Psychiatric patients have specific and general rights. The specific rights can vary from state to state. Rights of institutionalized patients are established by the state statutes and vary greatly. In general, patients have the right to:

- Adequate treatment, which includes:
  - a humane psychological and physical environment,
  - qualified personnel to provide individualized care, and
  - individualized treatment plans.
  - The right to be released if not dangerous.
  - The right to aftercare.

Some basic rights typically covered by statute are:
- Issues of confidentiality.
- Issues of involuntary detention.
- Right to send and receive mail.
- Right to consult with personal physician, attorney, or clergy.
- Rights of visitation unless documented reasons for denial.
- Rights to use personal possessions unless documented reasons for denial.
- Right to privacy and private storage space.
- Right to treatment in the least restrictive manner.
- Right to refuse treatment or medication.

- Right to refuse psychosurgery or electroconvulsive therapy (ECT).
- Right to receive help from patient advocates.

Patients are protected from strip and search except when valid consent is obtained or when there is adequate justification under the circumstances. Any time strip and search is done, it must be documented as a denial of rights stating why it was done.

Any time any of these rights are denied, there must be a sound reason and it must be documented. Denial of rights can never be punitive.

### Informed Consent

In most states patients must give written permission to be given psychotropic medications, except in an emergency and on a one-time basis. Patients must give informed consent to receive ECT. Patients must sign and understand a written informed consent to participate in any research protocols. They can never unknowingly participate in research. Voluntarily hospitalized patients must sign consent for treatment at the time of admission. Involuntary patients cannot give this consent.

### Confidentiality

Confidentiality is an important aspect of care for the psychiatric patient. There are state and hospital-specific laws, policies, and procedures. Patients have the right for no one to know that they are in a psychiatric facility. Be fully aware of your state and facility's laws and policies. Typically, upon admission patients are asked to sign a form stating what information they are willing to have shared if someone inquires about them.

There are times when confidentiality may be violated. If a patient is an imminent threat to himself or others, then confidentiality can be broken. Patients need to be told this before entering into a therapeutic relationship. If a patient makes a threat to harm a specific individual, the mental health professional must notify that individual per the Tarasoff law. If the health professional suspects physical, sexual, or financial abuse, he or she must report it to the appropriate authority.

### Involuntary Detentions

Individuals can be involuntarily committed for a psychiatric evaluation for only three reasons.
- They are a danger to themselves due to a mental illness.
- They are a danger to others due to a mental illness.
- They are gravely disabled due to a mental illness.

An involuntary detention can be placed by a police officer, a psychiatrist, or other designees appointed by the state. In some states, a psychiatric nurse clinician has this authority.

An initial hold is placed for up to 72 hours. During that time, only a psychiatrist can discontinue it. If the individual is still considered a danger to himself or others or is gravely disabled, he can be placed on an additional 14-day certification, but a court hearing must be held to uphold this. There are longer involuntary detentions in certain situations, such as a danger to others.

Individuals who are chronically mentally ill and unable to care for themselves may be given a conservator. This is someone who is appointed to make their decisions for them and who has the authority over individual and/or finances.

These laws vary from state to state.

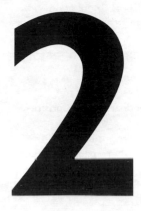

# Psychotherapeutic Theories

## Erikson's Eight Stages of Man

Erik Erikson defines man's growth and development from birth through old age. Each stage of development involves a MAJOR developmental task. This task must be achieved for a healthy transition to the next phase of development. Chapter 7 of *Childhood and Society* reviews these stages. Peck adds further concepts regarding stages seven and eight whose goals are generativity and ego integrity (Erikson, 1963).

### Stage One: Trust vs. Mistrust

*Birth to 1 year.*
- Corresponds to Freud's sensory/oral stage of development.
- Trust is defined by Webster as "… the assured reliance on another's integrity."
- Infant has to develop security in being cared for.
- Needs consistency and identification with the mother figure.
- Infant is dependent, passive, and has low frustration tolerance.
- Needs must be met for basic core of trust to develop.

### Stage Two: Autonomy vs. Shame and Doubt

*1–3 years of age.*
- Corresponds to Freud's anal/muscular stage of development.
- Child learning sense of self.
- Learning control over bodily functions; holding on and letting go; what is his and what is someone else's; where he begins and ends. *"toilet training"* *"it is my toy."*
- Learning limits and what is permissible.
- Task is for child to learn these things and parent to teach these things successfully and without excessive shame or doubt.
- Autonomy = sense of rightful dignity and lawful independence.
- Shame = self-consciousness, one is visible and not ready to be visible; being "shamed" leads to repressed rage and defiance.
- Doubt = brother of shame; fear of being attacked or overpowered.

*moral development at 2½*

## Stage Three: Initiative vs. Guilt

*3–6 years of age.*
- Corresponds to Freud's genital/phallic/Oedipal stage of development.
- Guilt = sense of badness.
- Task of identification with same-sex parent to make oneself endearing to opposite-sex parent, natural seductiveness.
- To learn not to overmanipulate and to have a sense of moral responsibility.
- Natural sexual curiosity needs to be satisfied; questions about where babies come from and masturbation normal.
- Parents have to teach children what is appropriate without inflicting sense of badness about themselves, sex or their bodies.

## Stage Four: Industry vs. Inferiority

*6–12 years of age.*
- Corresponds to Freud's latency stage of development.
- "Entrance into life."
- Development of *multiple* skills.
- Experience success and failure.
- Manual and social dexterity.
- Need good role models outside the family, e.g., teachers, Scout leaders.
- To avoid a sense of inferiority, child must be exposed to multiple arenas to discover his or best skills.
- "Hero worship" and same-sex crushes common.

## Stage Five: Identity vs. Role Confusion

*12–18 years of age; puberty and adolescence.*
- "Who am I … rapper, skater, artist, druggie, nerd, retro?"
- Emancipation from parents and development of independence.
- Definition of sexual identity and role; straight, gay, popular, sexy.
- Gangs and cliques prevail; need for sense of belonging.
- Conflict of biological readiness for sexual expression vs. cultural conventions and need for more emotional maturity.
- Developing their ideology, morals, and values.

## Stage Six: Intimacy vs. Isolation

*Young adulthood.*
- Freud was asked what a normal individual should be able to do well. He answered, "To love and to work."
- Mate selection.
- Development of interests into creative work.
- Develop competencies.
- Solidify one's sexuality.
- Ability to make and keep a commitment.
- "Utopia of genitalia": mutuality of orgasm with a loved partner of the opposite sex with whom one is able and willing to share a mutual trust and with whom one is able and willing to regulate the cycles of work, procreation, and recreation so as to secure all the stages of a satisfactory development for the offspring.

## Stage Seven: Generativity vs. Stagnation

*Adulthood.*

- Stagnation = self-absorption.
- Establishing and guiding the next generation.
- Procreation.
- Man needs to be needed.
- Productivity and creativity.
- Man's relationships to his production and his progeny.
- Not all parents necessarily achieve generativity; one can achieve it without procreating.

## Peck further adds

- Valuing wisdom vs. physical powers.
- Socializing vs. sexualizing in human relationships.
- Emotional flexibility vs. impoverishment.
- Mental flexibility vs. mental rigidity.

## Stage Eight: Ego Integrity vs. Despair

*Maturity/old age.*

- Life review.
- Despair = fear of death.
- Balancing activity with withdrawal.
- Form new relationships to replace losses.
- Acceptance of changing role in family.
- Completing the parental role.
- "Acceptance of one's one-and-only life cycle as something that had to be and that by necessity, permitted of no substitutions."
- Trust = "… the assured reliance on another's integrity." "Healthy children will not fear life if their elders have integrity enough not to fear death."

## Peck further delineates:

- Ego differentiation vs. work-role preoccupation. Establishment of valued activities and new roles to modify loss of occupation and parental role.
- Body transcendence vs. body preoccupation. Stress ability to focus on comforts, enjoyments, and mental tasks while de-emphasizing body aches, pains, and losses.
- Ego transcendence vs. ego preoccupation. Stresses living usefully and placing more value on what has been accomplished and what will be left behind for children and society rather than concentrating on personal death.

## Maslow's Hierarchy of Needs

### Self Actualization

Fulfillment of one's unique potential, personal growth and maturity, increased creativity and decreased conventionality.

### Love and Belonging

Acceptance of oneself, giving and receiving affection, identification with a group, warm relationships.

### Esteem

Sense of value and usefulness, self esteem and the respect of others, success in work, prestige.

### Safety Needs

Protection from harm, freedom from pain, stability, a predictable world order, attaining security.

### Physiological Needs

Water, food, oxygen, circulation, waste elimination, normal temperature, sleep, sexual expression.

**One cannot proceed to the next level until the prior levels are met.**
**When prioritizing nursing care, move up the hierarchy from physiological needs.**

# Seyle's Stress Theory

> *Complete freedom from stress is death.*
> —Hans Seyle

Hans Seyle defines **stress** as: "The nonspecific response of the body to any demand made upon it." Stress can be nervous tension, physical injury, infection, cold, heat, x-ray, or anything else. **Stressors** are any stimuli that the individual perceives as challenging, threatening, or demanding. They can be biological, psychological, or sociocultural. Stressors can be internal or external. Seyle further defines **eustress** as "good" stress. This is the stress of life that is coped with and can stimulate an individual to try new and more effective ways of adapting (Seyle, 1956).

Stress adaptation theory describes a **general adaptation syndrome**. It is general because it is produced only by agents that have a general effect upon large portions of the body. Adaptive means it stimulates defenses and thereby helps in the acquisition and maintenance of a stage of inurement (to make accustomed to something difficult or painful). The syndrome's manifestations are coordinated and partly dependent upon each other. The three stages are:

## Stage I — Stage of Alarm

The function of the stage of alarm is to mobilize the body's defensive forces. Physical manifestations of the alarm stage are marked loss of body weight, increase in hormone levels, and enlargement of the adrenal cortex and lymph glands. Psychological manifestations follow a pattern. First, the individual is alerted to stress, then the level of anxiety increases. The individual then moves into task-oriented and defense-oriented behavior. Symptoms of maladjustment, such as anxiety and ineffective behavior, may appear.

## Stage II — Stage of Resistance

The function of this stage is to achieve optimal adaptation to stress. Physical manifestations may include weight returning to normal, lymph glands returning to normal size, reduction in the size of adrenal cortex, and constant hormonal levels. Psychological manifestations of a individual in this stage are intensified use of coping mechanisms. The individual in this phase tends to use habitual defenses rather than problem-solving behavior. Psychosomatic symptoms may appear. If this stage is prolonged and coping and defenses are not effective, the individual will move into exhaustion.

*using drug alcohol*

## Stage III — Stage of Exhaustion

The body resources are depleted and the organism loses the ability to resist stress. Physical manifestations are weight loss, enlargement and depletion of adrenal glands, enlargement of lymph glands, and destruction of the lymphatic system. An increase in hormone levels and subsequent hormonal depletion also occurs. If excessive stress continues, the individual may die. Psychological manifestations of a individual in the stage of exhaustion are personality disorganization and a tendency toward exaggerated and inappropriate use of defense mechanisms. He or she may also exhibit an increased disorganization of thought and perceptions. The individual may lose contact with reality

*Epi / Non-Epi*
*immu system*

and delusions and hallucinations may appear. Further exposure to stress may result in complete psychological disintegration. Patients with chronic Posttraumatic Stress Disorder (PTSD) are physically debilitated, more prone to diseases, and psychologically unable to cope with normal amounts of stress.

Seyle also defines **local adaptation syndrome**. This is the manifestation of stress in a limited part of the body, an infected wound, for example. The same stages of adaptation apply.

The symptoms of damaging stress are exhibited biologically and psychologically. Not all symptoms are present in every individual. Physically the individual can exhibit elevated blood levels of adrenalines, corticoids, and ACTH. The eosinophil rate can drop. Elevated cholesterol and fatty acids may be present as well as elevated blood pressure and heart rate. Changes in EEG activity can be seen. Galvanic skin response shows changes. Other symptoms such as dry mouth, fatigue, trembling, accident proneness, insomnia, sweating, polyuria, GI distress, headaches, disruption of menstrual cycle, pain, and anorexia are often exhibited.

Psychological signs and symptoms of stress include anxiety symptoms such as irritability, hyperexcitation, hyperkinesis, nervous laughter, free-floating anxiety, hyperalertness, and an exaggerated startle reflex. Depressive symptoms are often present. The individual may have an overpowering urge to cry or run and hide and shows a loss of enjoyment in life. Nightmares are common. Substance abuse may occur or be exacerbated if already present. Cognition can be affected and be exhibited by an inability to concentrate, memory lapses, flight of thoughts, and/or disorientation. Psychosis may occur.

## Life Change Index Scale

Holmes and Rahe (1967) developed a Life Change Index Scale to determine stress levels. They define life change units (LCUs) and use a numerical scale of changes in one's life, both positive and negative, to score a individual's risk for damaging stress. The higher the score, the more prone the individual is to have a change in health status. This can be a predictor of a relapse into a preexisting condition, such as alcoholism, schizophrenia, or cancer.

According to the Life Change Index Scale, the top 10 life events are:
1. death of spouse
2. divorce
3. marital separation
4. jail term
5. death of close family member
6. personal illness or injury
7. marriage
8. fired at work
9. marital reconciliation
10. retirement

As these events occur, stress management becomes critical. Coping mechanisms are responses that arise as potentially stressful experiences occur. Problem solving is externally focused. Knowing how patients cope and teaching them to broaden their repertoire is good therapy.

Defense mechanisms are internal, often unconscious ways an individual copes with stress and life in general. They are presented separately in this manual. Assist the patient to shift from destructive to constructive defense mechanisms.

Stressor avoidance is the concept of foresight and planning. This is helping the patient to learn to avoid stressors when possible. An example would be avoiding situations that have been known to trigger panic attacks in the past. Assisting the patient to learn what triggers his/her stress reaction is also very important.

Conflict resolution is a useful tool. Deal with the stressor and resolve it if possible. This goes along with other forms of stress removal, such as changing jobs or getting divorced when necessary.

Learning to resist stress is also important. Mental preparation can help a individual learn to control the meaning of the situation before it can elicit a stress response. Physical preparation to prepare for stressful periods is wise. This includes nutrition, exercise, and rest. Another way to prepare is to gather information and to be intellectually prepared. Attitude changes and creative boosts can also help a individual be more resistant to a stressful event or period.

Employing stress reduction techniques when stressed is very important. Cognitive restructuring can help to control the stress reaction after it has developed. Relaxation responses such as meditation, prayer, and breathing exercises are very valuable. Spirituality is a great strength to draw upon. Sleep is, of course, vital and should be addressed. Exercise is a powerful stress reliever.

The more stress one is under, the more social support one needs: "We heal in community." Patients should be encouraged to seek out and expand social supports during periods of stress. This helps the supporter as well as the individual being supported and fulfills the need for a sense of belonging. Encourage patients to seek the help they need when stressed, whether it is in the form of emotional support or physical support.

## General Systems Theory

General systems theory is a most useful theory because it can be applied broadly. Two of the major theorists are Ludwig von Bertalanffy (1968) and Kurt Lewin (1935). A system can be an individual, a family, a hospital or institution, a unit within an institution, or the world.

A system is a set of parts meshing with each other within a **boundary**. There are **inputs**, **outputs**, and **throughputs** across this boundary. Certain basic premises apply to any system. One is that a phenomenon cannot be understood independently of the system of which it is a part. Another premise is that an impact on one component of a system affects the functioning of the total system. The natural drive of a system is to achieve steady state. **Equilibrium** is the balance among the parts of the system. **Steady state** is when there is a balanced relationship among all the components of a system. However, within the system, there are two opposing forces—one produces change and the other tends to halt change. Therefore, change of a system takes time and the correct amount of force to maintain equilibrium as the change is taking place.

All living systems are **open systems**, with contacts across boundaries with input, output, and a functional feedback system. **Feedback** is another key feature of systems theory. Systems maintain function and balance through communication. The message requires a sender and a receiver. The nature of the message sent determines how the return message will be structured or how long the interchange will last. An individual is an open system in a state of constant exchange with other individuals and the environment. Strictly defined, no systems are truly closed, but a given system may have minimal inputs and outputs for a while. This can be where the interventions/treatments nurses and other health care providers render are applied.

## Psychoanalytical Theory

Psychoanalysis is the moving of information from the unconscious to the conscious. It is the removal of amnesia, the recovery of repressed memories, and the interpretation of resistance. The goal of the therapy is to strengthen the ego and to decrease inner conflict. Sigmund Freud and Carl Jung are the two main authors of this theory of personality.

### Freud

Freud developed the concept of psychosexual stages of development and that symptoms occur due to regression or fixation on one of these psychosexual stages. Freud also defined the personality as consisting of three major systems: the id, the ego, and the superego. Discordant interaction among the three systems can lead to maladjusted behavior. The id functions on a primitive level and houses instinctual drives and psychic energy (libido). The ego is the aspect of the personality that is in contact with reality. The ego's primary function is to mediate between the instinctual impulses and the environment. The superego develops when the individual has the capacity to identify with and internalize the prohibitions and demands of parent figures. It includes the conscience. The superego evolves in response to rewards and punishments. The superego can be in conflict with the id and ego as it fulfills its functions of inhibiting the expression of id impulses, persuading the ego to substitute moralist goals for realistic ones, or strives for perfection. Freud's stages of development are described in the table below (Freud, 1959):

| Stage | Age | Developmental Task |
|---|---|---|
| Oral | birth to 18 months | Establishment of trusting dependence. |
| Anal | 18 months to 3 years | Development of self-control, feeling of autonomy. |
| Phallic | 3–5 years | Establishment of sexual identity. |
| Latency | 6–12 years | Group identification. |
| Prepuberty & Adolescence | 12–15 years | Development of social control over instincts. |
| Genital | 15 years to adult | Resolution of dependence-independence conflict. |

### Jung

Carl Jung further describes the role of the unconscious as a determinant of behavior. He defines the **personal unconscious** as the individual's experiences that were once conscious but have been transformed by repression, suppression, or other mechanisms. The **collective unconscious** is the inherited, racial foundation of the personality. It is a residue of the individual's evolutionary development, an accumulation of experiences passed down by ancestors. **Archetypes** are symbols derived from the collective unconscious.

The concepts of **anima** and **animus** relate to the essentially bisexual nature of individuals. The anima is the female archetype and the animus is the masculine archetype. Each individual contains both within their personality structure. The **shadow** archetype represents the unacceptable parts of one's personality. Acceptance of one's shadow and the shadow's tendencies moves one towards a wholeness of personality (Jung, 1966).

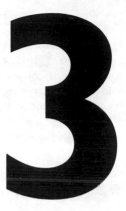

# Assessment and Diagnosis

## Psychiatric Assessment and Evaluation

### The Nursing Process

Before beginning any interaction with a patient, it is useful to remember the nursing process—assess, plan, implement, and evaluate. A nurse must perform an assessment before she can decide what to do. Assessment skills are vital. Only when a nursing diagnosis or medical diagnosis is obtained can appropriate care be planned. When planning for the patient's care, several factors must be considered.

The diagnosis is first, then the nurse must draw upon theoretical frameworks and reason out what should be done, taking into account available resources. There is a rationale for this sequence. An implementation you think is appropriate may not be available or the patient may not be willing to cooperate with that particular intervention. The nurse must then go back to redefining the problem and begin again.

Evaluation is an important part of the process. This is how a nurse decides if interventions were effective and appropriate and strategizes for an even better process next time in a similar situation.

The goals of a psychiatric assessment are varied. One is to collect a valid database from which to work. From that database, a tentative diagnosis can be made and an appropriate disposition and treatment plan can be determined. Another is to establish a sound engagement of the patient in the therapeutic alliance. During the process the nurse wants to develop an evolving and compassionate understanding of the patient, decrease the patient's anxiety, and instill hope. These factors help to ensure that the client will return for care (Shea, 1998).

There are many levels of psychiatric evaluation—from a very quick emergency evaluation where immediate intervention is required to a full diagnostic workup in an outpatient clinic. Some or all of the following information is necessary to obtain. Ideally, cooperation and rapport are attained before the interview. Whatever the situation, try to make the patient feel as comfortable as possible. Be respectful of the patient's right to privacy and put him or her at ease. A patient's history is a good predictor of the future. Take the time to obtain an adequate history whenever possible. Prior treatment providers, family members, and friends are often needed to supply information. This can be done in an appropriately confidential and ethical manner, as with any other type of illness. Keep the bio-psycho-social model in mind. Rule out physical causation before assigning psychiatric causation. Some diagnoses are more complex than others to ascertain and often patients have multiple diagnoses—some medical, some social, and some psychiatric. The sequence of the assessment may vary depending on many factors. Also, keep in mind that in most situations this is an ongoing assessment over time.

## Interview Process and Data Gathering

- **Identifying Information:** Name, Age, Sex, Race/Ethnicity, Marital Status, Religion, Language spoken.
- **Presenting Problem/Chief Complaint:** Patient's or family member's subjective statement of reason for being there. Why now?
- **Appearance:**
  - Description of individual: height, weight, grooming.
  - Unusual behaviors: Avoids eye contact, tremors, ambulation difficulties, tics, hyperactivity, speech abnormalities, somnolence, and intoxication. (Explain the reason for the interview, what is expected of them, how long this will take, and what will happen next. Explain that some questions may not apply to them.)
- **History:**
  - Psychiatric Illness:
    - Prior hospitalizations. When? Why?
    - Other treatments: group, individual, what worked, what did not work?
    - Diagnoses given.
    - Past psychiatric medications:
      - What meds worked.
      - Side effects and adverse reactions to medications.
      - Assess for tardive dyskinesia if patient has been or is on neuroleptics.
    - Current psychiatric medications:
      - Exact dosages prescribed and what the patient is actually taking. If on lithium, carbamazepine or valproic acid: date and result of last blood level.
  - Substance Abuse disorders and treatment:
    - Evidence of intoxication: postpone interview if possible if individual intoxicated.
    - Get drug toxicity screen if possible.
    - Has patient been treated in a substance abuse program?
    - Family history of alcoholism or drug abuse.
    - Continue if you still suspect substance use.
    - Attendance at 12-step meetings?
    - Current usage:
      - Alcohol:
        - Last drink. Be alert for potential withdrawal.
        - Drinking pattern.

- How many times per week does individual drink?
- How many times per week does individual drink to intoxication?
- Drugs:
  - Last use and what?
  - What substances used and frequency of use: speed, heroin, cocaine, sedatives, and marijuana? IV use?
- Do you think your alcohol or drug use is a problem?
- Family history:
  - Genogram.
  - Sexual abuse.
  - Physical abuse or neglect.
  - History of mental illness or alcoholism in the family.

## Mental Status Exam:

- Attitude toward examiner: cooperative, hostile, guarded.
- Speech: poverty of speech, poverty of content, pressured/rapid, slurred.
- Mood:
  - Depressed: increased or decreased sleep, increased or decreased weight, fatigue, energy level, anhedonia, interest, concentration.
  - Manic or hypomanic: hyperverbal, grandiose, sleeplessness, hypersexual, poor financial decisions, euphoric or irritable.
  - Anxious. Panic attacks.
  - Irritable.
  - Angry.
- Affect:
  - Inappropriate.
  - Flat.
  - Constricted.
  - Labile.
  - Normal: full range of appropriate emotional expression.
- Suicidal/Homicidal potential:
  - Current suicidal ideas/plans.
  - Past suicide attempts and details. Method, lethality, when, what interventions were taken at the time.
  - Current homicidal ideas/plans. Be aware of Tarasoff law.
  - Past incidents of harming others/spouse/children (outside of combat).
  - History of destroying property.
- Perception: Specify content.
  - Hallucinations.
    - Visual—often has organic cause.

- Auditory—more common in psychiatric illness.
- Command hallucinations.
- Thought content: Specify content.
  - Delusions.
  - General suspiciousness/paranoia.
  - Depersonalization: apart from under the influence of substances.
  - Dissociation.
- Thought process: Specify content.
  - Tangential.
  - Circumstantial.
  - Flight of thought.
  - Thought blocking.
- OCD Screening. Especially for patients with symptoms of anxiety.
  - Obsessions: Do you have repeated thoughts that you cannot get out of your head?
  - Compulsions: Do you ever feel compelled to do certain things over and over for no reason? Do you feel an emotional release after performing your ritualistic behavior? How much does this behavior interfere with your daily functioning?
- Cognitive Screening: Nonpsychotic patients failing one or more of these sections may need formal neuropsychological evaluation for dementia.
  - Intermediate-term memory: Recalls 3 of 4 words after 3–5 minutes of interviewing.
  - Orientation: Person. Place. Time.
  - Attention: Able to repeat 4 digits forward.
  - Concentration: Able to repeat 4 digits backwards.
  - Calculations: e.g., calculate 5 x 13, or, if unable, 19 + 8.
  - Verbal abstraction: e.g., how are an orange and a banana alike (fruit, food)?
  - General Information: How many weeks in a year? Where does the sun rise?
- Judgment and Insight: Inferred from history and observations.

## Medical Assessment:

- Current medical problems.
- Past major medical problems.
- Treatment providers, past and present.
- Surgeries.
- History of head trauma.
- Sleep patterns.
- Seizures.
- Last physical exam.
- Current medications.
- Allergies and adverse reactions.

## Social Assessment:

- Living situation.
- Social support system. Friends. Family. Church.
- Income. Financial resources.
- Legal considerations:
  - Conservatorship/payee.
  - Arrests, including DUI, public intoxication, and drug selling/possession.
  - Jail/prison history.
  - Current legal issues: parole, probation, charges pending, upcoming court dates.
- Education.
- Employment: current and past employment and job skills.
- Marital history; children.
- Military history:
  - Branch of service, dates of service, job, rank, type of discharge.
  - Service-connected disabilities (when illness first appears while in the military).
  - Past combat and wounds from such.
  - Sexual harassment or assault.
  - Evidence of PTSD.
  - Treatment for PTSD.

At this point additional tools, screenings, or diagnostic testing may be used. The Beck Depression Inventory is a quick, self-administered tool. Perform the Abnormal Involuntary Movement Scale Exam if the patient has been or is currently on neuroleptic agents to assess for tardive dyskinesia. If the diagnosis is still unclear, further medical or psychological testing may be indicated.

Using all the above information, you are ready to formalize your assessment and diagnose or define the patient's problem(s). At that time a plan for treatment and intervention is appropriate (Wilson & Kniesel, 1996; Beck, Rawlins, & Williams, 1993).

# Diagnostics and Disease-Specific Treatments

## Diagnostic and Statistical Manual of Mental Disorders IV, Text Revision

The DSM-IV-TR is the *Diagnostic and Statistical Manual of Mental Disorders, Fourth Edition, Text Revision,* published by the American Psychiatric Association in 2000. It is a classification of mental disorders with incidence, symptomatology, and gender differences. The purpose of the DSM-IV-TR is to provide clear descriptions of diagnostic categories to enable clinicians and investigators to diagnose, communicate about, study, and treat individuals with mental illnesses. The DSM-IV-TR focuses on clinical work, research, and education. It is supported by an extensive empirical foundation. The highest priority was to provide a helpful guide to clinical practice. DSM-IV-TR text contains a culture-specific section, a glossary of culture-bound syndromes, and the provision of an outline for cultural formulation. These are designed to enhance the cross-cultural use of the DSM-IV-TR. The DSM-IV-TR codes and terms are fully compatible with the codes and terms of ICD-10.

Since it is beyond the scope of this work to include all diagnostic criteria and categories, this section will cover broad concepts and partial descriptors of the illnesses. Only the most frequently encountered mental illnesses for adults will be addressed. Please refer to the DSM-IV-TR for complete information. Childhood disorders and pervasive developmental disabilities will not be covered.

## Multiaxial Assessment

The multiaxial system provides a convenient format for organizing and communicating clinical information. It brings attention to the various mental disorders and general medical conditions. It includes the psychosocial and environmental problems and describes the level of functioning.

There are five axes included in the DSM-IV-TR multiaxial classification:

Axis I    Clinical Disorders (psychiatric Disorders)
          Other Conditions That May Be a Focus of Clinical Attention
Axis II   Personality Disorders ) not treatable / Insurance won't pay.
          Mental Retardation
Axis III  General Medical Conditions
Axis IV   Psychosocial and Environmental Problems
Axis V    Global Assessment of Functioning

Axis I is for reporting all the various disorders or conditions in the classification except for Personality Disorders and Mental Retardation. These are reported on Axis II. If more than one Axis I disorder is present, the principal diagnosis or the reason for the visit should be listed first.

Axis II is for reporting Personality Disorders and Mental Retardation. Axis II may also be used to indicate prominent maladaptive personality features that do not meet the threshold for a Personality Disorder. The habitual use of maladaptive defense mechanisms may also be indicated.

Axis III is for reporting current general medical conditions that are potentially relevant to the understanding or management of the individual's mental disorder. When a mental disorder is judged a direct physiological consequence of the general medical condition, a Mental Disorder Due to a General Medical Condition should be diagnosed on Axis I and the general medical condition should be recorded on both Axis I and Axis III.

Axis IV describes the stressors causing Psychosocial and Environmental Problems that may affect the diagnosis, treatment, and prognosis of mental disorders that are listed on Axes I and II. Several areas may need to be addressed, such as:

• Problems with primary support group include the death of a family member, separation, divorce or estrangement, removal from the home, and remarriage of a parent. Sexual/physical abuse, parental overprotection, neglect, or discord with siblings, including birth of a sibling, should also be noted.

• Problems related to the social environment could include death/loss of a friend, inadequate social support/living alone, difficulty with acculturation/discrimination, and adjustment to life cycle transition.

- Education problems would include illiteracy or discord with teachers and classmates.
- Occupational problems would include unemployment, threat of job loss, stressful work schedule/conditions or job dissatisfaction, job change, or discord with the boss or coworkers.
- Housing problems would include homelessness or having inadequate housing or having discord with neighbors.
- Economic problems would include poverty, inadequate finances, or welfare support.
- Health care issues would include inadequate access to healthcare services.
- Legal related problems include arrest/incarceration, litigation, or being a crime victim.
- Other psychosocial and environmental problems may include exposure to disasters or hostilities.

*Axis V* is the Global Assessment of Functioning (GAF) scale is used to report the overall functioning of the patient. See table 3-1.

## Table 3-1. Global Assessment of Functioning (GAF) Scale

| | |
|---|---|
| 100 | Superior functioning in a wide range of activities, life problems never seem to get out of hand, and the individual is sought out by others because of his or her many positive qualities. No symptoms. |
| 90 | Absent or minimal symptoms (e.g., mild anxiety before an exam), good functioning in all areas, interested and involved in a wide range of activities, socially effective, generally satisfied with life, no more than everyday problems or concerns (e.g., an occasional argument with family members). |
| 80 | If symptoms are present, they are transient and expectable reactions to psychosocial stressors (e.g., difficulty concentrating after family argument): no more than slight impairment in social, occupational, or school functioning (e.g., temporarily falling behind in schoolwork). |
| 70 | Some mild symptoms (e.g., depressed mood and mild insomnia) OR some difficulty in social, occupational, or school functioning (e.g., occasional truancy, or theft within the household) but generally functioning pretty well, has some meaningful interpersonal relationships. |
| 60 | Moderate symptoms (e.g., flat affect and circumstantial speech, occasional panic attacks) OR moderate difficulty in social, occupational, or school functioning (e.g., few friends, conflicts with peers or coworkers). |
| 50 | Serious symptoms (e.g., suicidal ideation, severe obsessional rituals, frequent shoplifting) OR serious impairment in social, occupational, or school functioning (e.g., no friends, unable to keep a job). |
| 40 | Some impairment in reality testing or communication (e.g., speech is at times illogical, obscure, or irrelevant) OR major impairment in several areas, such as work or school, family relations, judgment, thinking, or mood (e.g., depressed man avoids friends, neglects family, and is unable to work; child frequently beats up younger children, is defiant at home, and is failing at school). |

*Table 3-1 continued.*

| | |
|---|---|
| 30 | Behavior is considerably influenced by delusions or hallucinations OR serious impairment in communication or judgment (e.g., sometimes incoherent, grossly inappropriate behavior, suicidal preoccupation) OR inability to function in almost all areas (e.g., stays in bed all day; no job, home, or friends). |
| 20 | Some danger of hurting self or others (e.g., suicide attempts without clear expectation of death; frequently violent; manic excitement) OR occasionally fails to maintain minimal personal hygiene (e.g., smears feces) OR gross impairment in communication (e.g., largely incoherent or mute). |
| 10 | Persistent danger of severely hurting self or others (e.g., recurrent violence) OR persistent inability to maintain minimal personal hygiene OR serious suicidal act with clear expectation of death. |
| 0 | inadequate information |

*Not Otherwise Specified.* It is impossible for diagnostic nomenclature to cover every possible situation. Each diagnostic class has at least one Not Otherwise Specified (NOS) category. There are four situations in which a NOS diagnosis may be appropriate:

• Presentation conforms to general guidelines for a mental disorder, but the symptomatic picture does not meet the criteria for any of the specific disorders.

• Presentation conforms to a symptom pattern that has not been included in the DSM-IV-TR classification but that causes clinically significant distress or impairment.

• There is uncertainty about etiology. The disorder may be due to a general medical condition, may be substance- induced, or may be primary.

• There is insufficient opportunity for complete data collection.

## Frequently Used Criteria

It is frequently necessary to include exclusion criteria to establish boundaries between disorders and to clarify differential diagnoses. Examples are:
• Criteria have never been met for …
• Criteria are not met for …
• Does not occur exclusively during the course of …
• Not due to the direct physiological effects of a substance or a general medical condition.

## Diagnostic Categories and Treatment Issues

*Schizophrenia and Other Psychotic Disorders and Treatments*
Schizophrenia is a disturbance that lasts for at least six months and includes at least one month of active-phase symptoms.

• Characteristic symptoms: Two or more of the following symptoms are present.
  • Delusions
  • Hallucinations
  • Disorganized speech
  • Grossly disorganized or catatonic behavior

- Negative symptoms (affective flattening, alogia, avolition)

  Note: Only one Criterion I symptom is required if delusions are bizarre or hallucinations consist of a voice keeping up a running commentary on the individual's behavior or thought or of two or more voices conversing with each other.

- Social/occupational dysfunction: For a significant portion of the time since the onset of the disturbance, one or more major areas of functioning such as work, interpersonal relations, or self-care are markedly below the level achieved prior to the onset.
- Duration: Continuous signs of the disturbance persist for at least 6 months.
- Schizoaffective and mood disorder exclusion: Schizoaffective disorder and mood disorder with psychotic features have been ruled out because either:
  - No major depressive, manic, or mixed episodes have occurred concurrently with the active-phase symptoms; or
  - if mood episodes have occurred during active-phase symptoms, their total duration has been brief relative to the duration of the active and residual periods.
- Substance/general medical condition exclusion: The disturbance is not due to the direct physiological effects of a substance or a general medical condition.
- Relationship to a pervasive developmental disorder: If there is a history of autistic disorder or another pervasive developmental disorder, the additional diagnosis of schizophrenia is made only if prominent delusions or hallucinations are also present for at least a month (or less if successfully treated).
  - Schizophrenia Subtypes: The subtypes of schizophrenia are defined by the predominant symptomatology at the time of evaluation.
    - Catatonic type is characterized by extreme psychomotor disruption, either reduced movement and negativism or active but purposeless movements not influenced by surroundings.
    - Disorganized type is characterized by disorganized speech and behavior and flat or inappropriate affect.
    - Paranoid type is associated with preoccupation with delusions or frequent hallucinations. Hallucinations and delusions are persecutory or grandiose.
    - Undifferentiated type is assigned when a patient presents with prominent active phase symptoms not meeting criteria for the catatonic, disorganized, or paranoid type.
    - Residual type is for presentations in which there is continuing evidence of the disturbance, but the criteria for the active-phase symptoms are no longer met. Negative symptoms like flat affect and inability to work are present.
- Schizophreniform Disorder
  - The essential features of schizophreniform disorder are identical to those of schizophrenia (criterion I) except for two differences. The total duration of the illness is at least 1 month but less than 6 months and impaired social or occupational functioning during some part of the illness is not required. Schizophreniform disorder may be prodromal to schizophrenia or schizoaffective illness.
- Schizoaffective Disorder
  - The essential feature of schizoaffective disorder is an uninterrupted period of illness during which, at some time, there is either a major depressive episode, a

manic episode, or a mixed episode concurrent with symptoms that meet criterion I for schizophrenia.

- Other Psychotic Disorders
  - Delusional Disorder
  - Brief Psychotic Disorder
  - Shared Psychotic Disorder
  - Psychotic Disorder due to a general medical condition
  - Substance-induced Psychotic Disorder
  - Psychotic Disorder NOS
- Treatment for Schizophrenia and other Psychotic Disorders
  - Psychopharmacology: Antipsychotics
  - Case Management
  - Social Skills Training
  - Promoting Family Understanding and Involvement
  - Promoting Community Contacts

## Mood Disorders and Treatments

Mood disorders include disorders that have a disturbance in mood as the predominant feature.

- Major Depressive Episode
  - The essential feature of a major depressive episode is a period of at least 2 weeks during which there is either depressed mood or the loss of interest or pleasure in nearly all activities.
- Criteria for Major Depressive Episode
  - Five (or more) of the following symptoms have been present during the same 2-week period and represent a change from previous functioning: at least one of the symptoms is either 1) depressed mood or 2) loss of interest or pleasure.
    - Depressed mood most of the day, nearly every day, as indicated by either subjective report or observation made by others. (In children and adolescents, can be irritable mood.)
    - Markedly diminished interest or pleasure in all, or almost all, activities most of the day, nearly every day.
    - Significant weight loss when not dieting or weight gain, or decrease or increase in appetite nearly every day.
    - Insomnia or hypersomnia nearly every day.
    - Psychomotor agitation or retardation nearly every day that is observable by others, not merely subjective feelings of restlessness or being slowed down.
    - Fatigue or loss of energy nearly every day
    - Feelings of worthlessness or excessive or inappropriate guilt nearly every day.
    - Diminished ability to think or concentrate, or indecisiveness, nearly every day.
    - Recurrent thoughts of death, recurrent suicidal ideation without a specific plan, or a suicide attempt or a specific plan for committing suicide.

- The symptoms do not meet criteria for a mixed episode.
- The symptoms cause clinically significant distress or impairment in social, occupational, or other important areas of functioning.
- The symptoms are not due to the direct physiological effects of a substance or a general medical condition.
- The symptoms are not better accounted for by bereavement.

- Manic Episode
  - A distinct period of abnormally and persistently elevated, expansive, or irritable mood, lasting at least 1 week (or any duration if hospitalization is necessary.)
  - During the period of mood disturbance, three (or more) of the following symptoms have persisted (four if the mood is only irritable) and have been present to a significant degree:
    - inflated self-esteem or grandiosity
    - decreased need for sleep (e.g., feels rested after only 3 hours of sleep)
    - more talkative than usual or pressure to keep talking
    - flight of ideas or subjective experience that thoughts are racing
    - distractibility (e.g., attention too easily drawn to unimportant or irrelevant external stimuli)
    - increase in goal-directed activity (either socially, at work or school, or sexually) or psychomotor agitation
    - excessive involvement in pleasurable activities that have a high potential for painful consequences (e.g., engaging in unrestrained buying sprees, sexual indiscretions, or foolish business investments)
  - The symptoms do not meet criteria for a mixed episode.
  - The mood disturbance is sufficiently severe to cause marked impairment in occupational functioning or in usual social activities or relationships with others, or to necessitate hospitalization to prevent harm to self or others, or there are psychotic features.
  - The symptoms are not due to the direct physiological effects of a substance or a general medical condition.
- Mixed Episode: A period of time (lasting at least 1 week) in which the criteria are met both for a manic episode and for a major depressive episode nearly every day.
- Hypomanic Episode: A distinct period during which there is an abnormally and persistently elevated, expansive, or irritable mood that lasts at least 4 days.
- Dysthymic Disorder: A chronically depressed mood that occurs for most of the day more days than not for at least 2 years. It may be intermittent, with periods of feeling normal. These periods of relief last for no more than two months.
- Cyclothymic Disorder: Characterized by chronic, fluctuating mood disturbances involving numerous periods of hypomanic symptoms and numerous periods of depressive symptoms.
- Bipolar Disorders
  - Bipolar I Disorder is a clinical course that is characterized by the occurrence of one or more manic episodes or mixed episodes and episodes of major depression.

- Bipolar II Disorder is a clinical course that is characterized by the occurrence of one or more major depressive episodes accompanied by at least one hypomanic episode.

Note: Substance abuse is a frequent complication in all affective disorders.

Treatments for Bipolar Disorder
- Hospitalization
- Suicide prevention
- Biological treatments
  - Antidepressants for patients with depression:
    - SSRIs
    - Tricyclics
    - MAOIs
  - Mood stabilizers for patients with manic or hypomanic symptoms:
    - Lithium
    - Depakote
    - Tegretol
    - Gabapentine
  - Antipsychotics to treat psychotic symptoms.
    - Olanzapine (has indication for bipolar illness as well as psychosis)
    - Atypicals
    - Typicals
- Electroconvulsive therapy
- Individual Psychotherapy
- Group therapy
- Cognitive-behavioral therapy ⟹ *Boarderline personality*

## Cognitive Disorders and Treatments

Assessment for cognitive disorders is challenging because confused patients are often poor historians. Also, the interview environment and procedure may increase the individual's anxiety and compromise the assessment. Areas of subjective assessment include health history, sensory impairment, dietary history, history of head trauma, medication use, cognitive functioning, and overall mental status. Objective data include the physical examination, routine lab tests and scans, and objective scales of cognitive functioning.

*Delirium.* Delirium is a cognitive disorder characterized by global cognitive impairment of abrupt onset and relatively brief duration in which perception, thinking, and memory are all disrupted. It is common in adults and is usually caused by an underlying systemic illness. The goal of nursing interventions for patients with delirium is to support existing sensory perception until the client returns to previous levels of functioning. This is based on the premise that patients are capable of returning to their previous level of functioning. Maintaining optimal levels of sensory perception, participation in ADLs, and maintaining physiological homoeostasis during the period of the delirium are important. The most common forms of delirium, per DSM-IV-TR are:

- Delirium due to a General Medical Condition
- Substance-induced Delirium
- Delirium due to Multiple Etiologies
- Delirium NOS

*Dementia.* Dementia is marked by a loss of intellectual abilities of sufficient severity to interfere with social and occupational functioning. The goal of nursing interventions for patients with dementia is minimizing the loss of self-care capacity. Dementia involves progressive intellectual, behavioral, and physiological deterioration. Helping the family to sustain rewarding relationships throughout this terminal process is an important care component. Types of dementia, per DSM-IV-TR, are:

*Dementia of the Alzheimer's Type.* Alzheimer's disease is the most common form of dementia among the older adult. It is progressive, age-related, chronic dysfunction marked by phases: early phases of forgetfulness, more advanced phases of disorientation and diminished concentration, and later and terminal phases of severe agitation, disorientation, psychosis, and complete helplessness. Age, decreased levels of acetylcholine and serotonin, genetic factors, virus-like substances, and environmental toxins are all under consideration as possible causes. (Wilson & Kneisel, 1996). Acetylcholinesterase inhibitors such as donepexil (Aricept) are used to slow the cognitive decline of the patient with Alzheimer's disease. Other types of dementia identified by the DSM-IV-TR are:

- Vascular Dementia
- Other Dementias:
  - Dementia due to HIV Disease
  - Dementia due to Head Trauma
  - Dementia due to Parkinson's Disease
  - Dementia due to Huntington's Disease
  - Dementia due to Pick's Disease
  - Dementia due to Creutzfeldt-Jakob Disease
  - Dementia due to Other General Medical Conditions
    - Substance-induced
    - Multiple etiologies
    - NOS

## Anxiety Disorders and Treatments

Anxiety disorders are characterized by either recurrent or persistent psychological and physical symptoms that interfere with normal functioning, continue in the absence of obvious external stress, or are excessive responses to these stresses. Anxiety Disorders include:

- Panic Disorder
- Phobias
  - Agoraphobia
  - Specific Phobia
  - Social Phobia
- Generalized Anxiety Disorder
- Obsessive-Compulsive Disorder
- Acute Stress Disorder
- Post-traumatic Stress Disorder

*Panic Disorder.* The essential feature of panic disorder is the presence of recurrent, unexpected panic attacks, followed by at least 1 month of persistent concern about having another panic attack. A panic attack itself is not a codable disorder. Code the specific diagnosis in which the panic attack occurs (e.g., 300.21 Panic Disorder with Agoraphobia). A panic attack is a discrete period of intense fear or discomfort, in which four (or more) of the following symptoms develop abruptly and reach a peak within 10 minutes:

- palpitations, pounding heart, or accelerated heart rate
- sweating
- trembling or shaking
- sensations of shortness of breath or smothering
- feeling of choking
- chest pain or discomfort
- nausea or abdominal distress
- feeling dizzy, unsteady, lightheaded, or faint
- derealization (feelings of unreality) or depersonalization (being detached from oneself)
- fear of losing control or going crazy
- fear of dying
- paresthesias (numbness or tingling sensations)
- chills or hot flushes

*Panic Disorder without Agoraphobia* is characterized by recurrent unexpected panic attacks about which there is persistent concern.

*Panic Disorder with Agoraphobia* is characterized by both recurrent unexpected panic attacks and agoraphobia. Agoraphobia in this context means anxiety about, or avoidance of, places or situations from which escape might be difficult or embarrassing or in which help may not be available in the event of having a panic attack or panic-like symptoms.

Treatment of Panic Disorder
- Pharmacological:
  - Imipramine can prevent a high percentage of panic attacks.
  - Propranolol, a beta-adrenergic blocker, is particularly effective against somatic signs of anxiety. MAOIs can be effective for some cases of panic disorder, especially with agoraphobia.
  - SSRIs can be of some benefit for some patients.
  - Short-term use of anxiolytic agents has been proven effective, but should not be used long term.
- Behavioral Modification

## Phobic Disorders

*Agoraphobia* is the fear of being alone or in public places from which escape might be difficult or help might not be available. Agoraphobia is usually accompanied by panic attacks.

*Specific Phobia* is characterized by clinically significant anxiety provoked by a specific feared object or situation, often leading to avoidance behavior.

*Social Phobia* is characterized by clinically significant anxiety provoked by exposure to certain types of social or performance situations where the individual may be scrutinized. It often leads to avoidance behavior.

Treatments of Phobias
• Behavior Modification
• Systematic Desensitization

## Anxiety Disorders and Treatment

*Generalized Anxiety Disorder*
Diagnostic Criteria:
• Pervasive and persistent anxiety of at least 6 months duration without phobias, panic attacks, or obsessions and compulsions.
• Associated with mild depressive symptoms.
• Predisposed to the abuse of alcohol or other drugs.

Treatment of Generalized Anxiety Disorder
• Behavioral Therapy
• Individual Therapy

*Obsessive-Compulsive Disorder*
Obsessive-Compulsive Disorder is characterized by obsessions (which cause marked anxiety or distress) and/or by compulsions (which serve to neutralize anxiety). In obsession, the recurring thought cannot be dismissed from consciousness. In compulsion, there is an uncontrollable, persistent urge to perform certain acts or behaviors to relieve an otherwise unbearable tension.

Treatment of OCD
• Pharmacological
  • Anafranil (clomipramine) tricyclic antidepressant.
  • Prozac (fluoxetine) SSRI at high doses.
• Behavioral therapy

*Acute Stress Disorder*
The development of anxiety and dissociative symptoms occurring within 1 month of an extremely traumatic event. The precipitating stressors are similar to those of PTSD and include:

• Exposure to a traumatic event in which the individual experienced or witnessed event(s) that involved actual or threatened injury or death.
• A response involving helplessness, fear, or horror.
• Dissociative symptoms and avoidance of specific stimuli.
• Symptoms of hyperarousal.

Treatment of Acute Stress Disorder
• Critical incident debriefing.
• Short-term use of anxiolytics.
• Trauma victim support group.
• Individual therapy.

*Posttraumatic Stress Disorder*
• Acute: if duration of symptoms is less than 3 months.
• Chronic: if duration of symptoms is 3 months or more.
• With Delayed Onset: if onset of symptoms is at least 6 months after the stressor.

Diagnostic Criteria for PTSD
- The individual has been exposed to a traumatic event in which:
  - He or she experienced or witnessed an event that involved actual or threatened death or serious injury.
  - The individual's response involved intense fear, helplessness, or horror.
- The traumatic event is persistently re-experienced in one or more of the following ways:
  - Intrusive thoughts of the traumatic event.
  - Recurrent dreams of the traumatic event.
  - Feeling or acting as if the traumatic event were recurring.
  - Intense distress at exposure to internal or external cues that symbolize or resemble an aspect of the traumatic event.
  - Physiological reactivity on exposure to cues that symbolize or resemble an aspect of the traumatic event.
- The individual is engaged in persistent avoidance of stimuli associated with the trauma and experiences numbing of general responsiveness, as indicated by:
  - Efforts to avoid thoughts, feelings, or conversations associated with the trauma.
  - Efforts to avoid activities, places, or individuals that arouse recollections of the trauma.
  - Inability to recall an important aspect of the trauma.
  - Markedly diminished interest or participation in significant activities.
  - Restricted range of affect.
  - Sense of foreshortened future.
- Persistent symptoms of increased arousal are indicated by two or more of the following:
  - Difficulty falling or staying asleep.
  - Irritability or outbursts of anger.
  - Difficulty concentrating.
  - Hypervigilance.
  - Exaggerated startle response.
- Duration of the disturbance is more than 1 month.
- The disturbance causes clinically significant distress or impairment in social, occupational, or other important areas of functioning.

Prevalence and Causes of PTSD
- Causes
  - Sexual assault
  - Child abuse
  - Combat
  - Criminal assault
  - Natural disasters
  - Medical illnesses
  - Serious accidents
- Prevalence
  - 8% lifetime prevalence; 10% for women, 5% for men.
  - 2:1 women to men

- 60–80% of individuals will experience a traumatic event during their lifetime.
- 9% of women will be raped in their lifetime.
- Rape victims have a 50% incidence of PTSD.
- Vietnam veterans: 30% of men and 27% of the women who served have PTSD.

*Co-Morbid Conditions*
There is an increased risk of other disorders in individuals with Posttraumatic Stress Disorder. Often the patient has a concomitant illness. Some common co-morbid conditions are:
- Major depressive disorder: 50%
- Substance related disorders
- Panic disorder
- Agoraphobia
- Obsessive-compulsive disorder
- Social phobia
- Dissociative disorder

Treatment for Posttraumatic Stress Disorder
- Address possiblity of suicidal behavior.
- Address substance abuse.
- Group therapy.
- Individual therapy
- Education group.
- Psychopharmacology:
  - SSRIs to treat anxiety and depression.
  - Sleep issues: use Trazadone in combination with SSRI.

## Personality Disorders and Treatment
A personality disorder is an enduring, inflexible, pervasive pattern of inner experience and behavior that deviates markedly from the expectations of the individual's culture. The onset is during adolescence or early adulthood, continues over time, and leads to impairment and/or distress in social areas of functioning.

There are 10 types of personality disorders:
- Paranoid
- Schizoid
- Schizotypal
- Antisocial
- Borderline
- Histrionic
- Narcissistic
- Avoidant
- Dependent
- Obsessive-Compulsive

*Personality Disorder Not Otherwise Specified* is a category provided for two situations:

- The individual's personality pattern meets the general criteria for a personality disorder and traits of several different personality disorders are present, but the criteria for a specific personality disorder are not met; or

- The individual's personality pattern meets the general criteria for a personality disorder, but the individual is considered to have a personality disorder that is not included in the classification (e.g., passive-aggressive personality disorder).

Personality disorders are grouped into three clusters based on descriptive similarities (American Psychiatric Association, 2000):

*Cluster A:*  Paranoid, Schizoid, Schizotypal. Individuals may appear odd or eccentric

*Cluster B:*  Antisocial, Borderline, Histrionic, Narcissistic. Individuals often appear very dramatic, emotional, or erratic.

*Cluster C:*  Avoidant, Dependent, Obsessive-Compulsive Personality Disorder. Individuals with these disorders often appear anxious or fearful

The clustering system, although useful in some research and educational situations, has serious limitations. It has not been consistently validated. Individuals frequently present with co-occurring personality disorders from different clusters.

Shea, 1998, defined three broad groups of personality disorders that differ slightly from the DSM-IV-TR clustering system:
- Anxiety Prone Disorders (obsessive-compulsive, dependent, and avoidant)
- Poorly Empathic Disorders (schizoid, antisocial, histrionic, narcissistic)
- Psychotic Prone Personality Disorders (borderline, schizotypal, paranoid)

### Theories and Information about Personality Disorders
- Cluster B personality disorders (antisocial, borderline, histrionic, and narcissistic) are thought by some researchers to have a genetic base.
- Antisocial personality disorder is associated with alcohol use disorders.
- There is a strong association between histrionic personality disorder and somatization disorder.
- Cluster C personality disorders (avoidant, dependent, obsessive-compulsive, and NOS) may have a genetic base.
- Patients with avoidant personality disorder often have high anxiety levels.
- Patients with obsessive-compulsive personality disorder often show symptoms associated with depression.
- Individuals who exhibit impulsive traits also will often show increased levels of testosterone, 17-estradiol, and estrone.
- Androgens, in nonhuman primates, increase the likelihood of aggression and sexual behavior.
- Low levels of Monoamine Oxidase (MAO) have been associated with college students spending more time in social activities than students with high levels of MAO.
- Decreased serotonin causes depressive symptoms.
- Increase in dopamine causes euphoria.
- Slow-wave activity on EEGs is found most commonly in antisocial and borderline types.
- Some personality disorders may arise from poor parental fit (poor match between temperament and child-rearing practices).

- Cluster B disorders are associated with high levels of father educational involvement, father psychological maladjustment, high number of family stressors, low levels of maternal physical abuse, childhood sexual abuse, and poor paternal decision-making style.

*Personality traits* are an individual's enduring patterns of perceiving, relating to, and thinking of what is happening in their world and experience. A wide range of personal and social contexts are demonstrated. ONLY when personality traits are inflexible and maladaptive and cause significant functional impairment or subjective distress do they constitute personality disorders (American Psychiatric Association, 2000).

The patient with a personality disorder has impairment in functioning or subjective distress in at least two of the following areas:

- Criterion A:
  - Cognition (e.g., impairment in memory, decreased concentration)
  - Affectivity (e.g., emotional dysregulation)
  - Interpersonal functioning (e.g., inability to maintain friendships; inability to maintain coworker relationships causes individual to get fired from job)
  - Impulse control (e.g., spending sprees, binge drinking, binge eating)
- Criterion B:
  - This pattern is inflexible and pervasive across a variety of different situations (e.g., intense feelings of anger will follow them wherever they go).
- Criterion C:
  - This intense inner distress leads to a significant distress or impairment in social, occupational, or other important areas of functioning.
- Criterion D:
  - The pattern is stable and of long duration.
  - Onset can be traced back at least to adolescence or early adulthood.
- Criterion E:
  - The pattern is not accounted for as a manifestation or consequence of another mental disorder.
- Criterion F:
  - It is not due to the direct physiological effects of a substance or a medical condition.

## Documentation
Code personality disorders on Axis II:

- DSM-IV-TR suggests the listing of the defense mechanisms that the client uses.
- List all relevant personality disorder diagnoses in order of importance (when an individual's pattern of behavior meets criteria for more than one personality disorder).
- When an Axis I disorder is not the principal diagnosis or the reason for visit, indicate which personality disorder is the principal diagnosis.

## Anxiety Prone Personality Disorders
• Obsessive-Compulsive personality disorder.
• Dependent personality disorder.
• Avoidant personality disorder.

### Obsessive-Compulsive Personality Disorder

*Diagnostic Criteria.* A pervasive pattern of preoccupation with orderliness, perfectionism, and mental and interpersonal control, at the expense of flexibility, openness, and efficiency. This begins by early adulthood and is present in a variety of situations, as indicated by four (or more) of the following:

• Preoccupied with details, rules, lists, order, organization, or schedules to the extent that the major point of the activity is lost.

• Shows perfectionism that interferes with task completion

• Is excessively devoted to work and productivity to the exclusion of leisure activities and friendships.

• Is overconscientious, scrupulous, and inflexible about matters of morality, ethics, or values (not accounted for by cultural or religious identification).

• Is unable to discard worn-out or worthless objects even when they have no sentimental value (e.g., saves labels from water bottles).

• Is reluctant to delegate tasks or to work with others unless they submit to exactly his or her way of doing things.

• Adopts a miserly spending style toward both self and others; money is viewed as something to be hoarded for future catastrophes.

• Shows rigidity and stubbornness.

(American Psychiatric Association, 2000)

Prevalence of OCD Personality Disorder
• It affects 1% of individuals in community samples.
• It affects 3–10% of individuals presenting to mental health clinics.

Treatment of OCD Personality Disorder
• Group psychotherapy.
• Behavior therapy.
• SSRIs (fluoxetine usually at dosages of 60–80mg).

Differential Diagnoses
• Obsessive-Compulsive Disorder. Key is HOARDING is extreme in OCD.
• Narcissistic Personality Disorder. Obsessive-compulsive personality disorder is usually self-critical.
• Schizoid Personality Disorder. Schizoid has lack for capacity for intimacy.
• Personality change due to a general medical condition.
• Symptoms that may develop in association with chronic substance use.

## Dependent Personality Disorder

*Diagnostic Criteria.* A pervasive and excessive need to be cared for that leads to clinging and submissive behavior, with fears of separation. Begins by early adulthood and presents in a variety of contexts, including five (or more) of the following:

- Has difficulty making everyday decisions without an excessive amount of advice and reassurance from others.
- Needs others to assume responsibility for most major areas of his/her life.
- Has difficulty expressing disagreement with others because of fear of loss of support or approval.
- Has difficulty initiating projects or doing things on his/her own (due to lack of self-confidence in judgment or abilities rather than a lack of motivation or energy)
- Goes to excessive lengths to obtain nurturance and support from others, to the point of volunteering to do things that are unpleasant.
- Feels uncomfortable or helpless when alone because of exaggerated fears of being unable to care for himself/herself.
- Urgently seeks another relationship as a source of care and support when a close relationship ends.
- Is unrealistically preoccupied with fears of being left to take care of himself/herself.

(American Psychiatric Association, 2000).

*Prevalence of Dependent Personality Disorder:* Dependent personality disorder is among the most frequently reported personality disorders in mental health clinics.

Differential Diagnoses
- Dependency arising as a consequence of Axis I disorders, (e.g., mood disorders, panic disorder, agoraphobia) and as a result of a general medical condition.
- Dependent personality disorder has an early onset, chronic course, and a pattern of behavior that does not occur exclusively during an Axis I or Axis II disorder.
- Borderline personality disorder (individual with dependent personality disorder will react with increasing appeasement and submissiveness).
- Avoidant personality disorder (individuals will have a strong fear of humiliation and rejection so they withdraw until they are certain they will be accepted).

Treatment Strategies for Dependent Personality Disorder
- Individual psychotherapy
- Behavioral therapy
- Assertiveness training
- Family therapy
- Group therapy
- Pharmacotherapy: SSRIs to treat symptoms of anxiety and depression

## Avoidant Personality Disorder

*Diagnostic Criteria.* A pervasive pattern of social inhibition, feelings of inadequacy, and hypersensitivity to negative evaluation, beginning by early adulthood and present in a variety of contexts, as indicated by four (or more) of the following:

- Avoidance of occupational activities that require significant interpersonal contact, due to fears of criticism, rejection or disapproval.

- Unwillingness to get involved with individuals unless certain of being liked.
- Shows restraint within intimate relationships because of the fear of being shamed or ridiculed.
- Is preoccupied with being criticized or rejected in social situations.
- Inhibition in new interpersonal situations because of feelings of inadequacy.
- Views self as inferior to others, personally unappealing, and socially inept.
- Reluctant to take personal risks or to engage in new activities because they may prove embarrassing.

(American Psychiatric Association, 2000).

Differential Diagnoses
- There is a great amount of overlap between avoidant personality disorder and social phobia, generalized type.
- Avoidant personality disorder and panic disorder with agoraphobia often co-occur.

Treatment of Avoidant Personality Disorder
- Individual psychotherapy
- Social skills therapy
- Behavior therapy (e.g., assertiveness training).
- Pharmacotherapy:
  - Atenolol (Tenormin) a beta-blocker to manage autonomic nervous system hyperactivity.
  - SSRIs may help their rejection sensitivity.

## Poorly Empathic Personality Disorders
- Schizoid Personality Disorder
- Antisocial Personality Disorder
- Histrionic Personality Disorder
- Narcissistic Personality Disorder

*Schizoid Personality Disorder*
*Diagnostic Criteria.* A pervasive pattern of detachment from social relationships and a restricted range of expression of emotions in interpersonal settings, beginning by early adulthood and present in a variety of contexts, as indicated by four (or more) of the following:

- Neither desires nor enjoys close relationships, including being part of a family.
- Almost always chooses solitary activities.
- Has little, if any, interest in having sexual experiences with another individual.
- Experiences pleasure in few, if any, activities.
- Lacks close friends or confidantes other than first-degree relatives.
- Appears indifferent to the praise or criticism of others.
- Shows emotional coldness, detachment, or flattened affectivity.

*Does not occur exclusively during the course of schizophrenia, a mood disorder with psychotic features, another psychotic disorder, or a pervasive developmental disorder and is not due to the direct physiological effects of a general medical condition.*

Differential Diagnoses
- Delusional disorder
- Schizophrenia
- Mood disorder with psychotic features,

- Autistic disorders
- Personality change due to a general medical condition
- Symptoms that may develop in association with chronic substance use

Treatment of Schizoid Personality Disorder
- Group psychotherapy: work on issues of trust.
- Pharmacotherapy: small dosages of antipsychotics to clear thinking,
- Antidepressants to treat depression and anxiety.
- SSRIs may make patients less sensitive to rejection.

*Antisocial Personality Disorder*
Prevalence
- 3% in males and about 1% in females
- Varies between 3–30% in clinical settings
- There is a higher prevalence rate associated with substance abuse treatment settings and prison or forensic settings.
- Environmental and genetic factors contribute to the risk of this group.

Diagnostic Criteria for Antisocial Personality Disorder
- Pervasive pattern of disregard for and violation of the rights of others occurring since age 15 years, as indicated by three (or more) of the following:
  - Failure to conform to social norms with respect to lawful behaviors as indicated by repeatedly performing acts that are grounds for arrest.
  - Deceitfulness, as indicated by repeated lying, use of aliases, or conning others for personal profit or pleasure.
  - Impulsivity and aggressiveness, as indicated by repeated physical fights or assaults.
  - Reckless disregard for safety of self or others.
  - Consistent irresponsibility, as indicated by repeated failure to sustain consistent work behavior or honor financial obligations.
  - Lack of remorse, as indicated by being indifferent to or rationalizing having hurt, mistreated, or stolen from another.
- The individual is at least 18 years of age.
- Onset of conduct disorder is evident before age 15 years of age.
- Antisocial behavior does not occur exclusively during the course of schizophrenia or a manic episode.

(American Psychiatric Association, 2000).

Treatment of Antisocial Personality Disorder
- Psychotherapy
  - Establish firm limits.
  - Separate control from punishment.
  - Separate help and confrontation from social isolation and retribution.
- Pharmacotherapy
  - Psychostimulants (Ritalin) or Wellbutrin for co-existing ADHD.
  - Depakote to control impulsive behavior.

## Histrionic Personality Disorder

### Prevalence

- Diagnosed more frequently in females.
- Prevalent in about 2–3% of the general population.
- Noted in inpatient and outpatient health settings in 10–15% of the patient population.
- Noted with a tendency for somatization.

### Diagnostic Criteria

- A pervasive pattern of excessive emotionality and attention seeking, beginning by early adulthood and present in a variety of contexts, as indicated by five (or more) of the following:

  - Is uncomfortable in situations when he/she is not the center of attention.
  - Interaction with others is often characterized by inappropriate sexually seductive or provocative behavior.
  - Displays a rapidly shifting and shallow expression of emotions.
  - Consistently uses physical appearance to draw attention to self.
  - Has a style of speech that is excessively impressionistic and lacking in detail.
  - Shows self-dramatization, theatricality, and exaggerated expression of emotion.
  - Is suggestible; easily influenced by others or circumstances.
  - Considers relationships to be more intimate than they actually are.

(American Psychiatric Association, 2000).

### Treatment of Histrionic Personality Disorder

- Psychotherapy: Psychoanalytically-oriented therapy is the treatment of choice.
- Pharmacotherapy:
  - Antidepressants for depression and somatic complaints
  - Antianxiety agents for anxiety
  - Antipsychotics for derealization and illusions

## Narcissistic Personality Disorder

### Prevalence

- Narcissistic traits are particularly common in adolescents.
- Individuals may have difficulties adjusting to the onset of physical and occupational limitations that are inherent in the aging process.
- 50–75% of those diagnosed with this disorder are male.
- Prevalence ranges from 2–16% in the clinical population, less than 1% in the general population.

### Diagnostic Criteria

- A pervasive pattern of grandiosity (in fantasy or behavior), need for admiration, and lack of empathy, beginning by early adulthood and present in a variety of contexts, as indicated by five (or more) of the following:

  - Has a grandiose sense of self-importance (e.g., exaggerates achievement and talents, expects to be recognized as superior without commensurate achievements).

  - Is preoccupied with fantasies of unlimited success, power, brilliance, beauty, or ideal love.

  - Believes that he or she is "special" and unique and can only be understood by, or should associate with, other special or high-status individuals (or institutions).

- Requires excessive admiration.
- Has a sense of entitlement (e.g., unreasonable expectations of especially favorable treatment or automatic compliance with his/her expectations).
- Is interpersonally exploitive (e.g., takes advantage of others to achieve his/her own ends).
- Lacks empathy, is unwilling to recognize or identify with the feelings and needs of others.
- Is often envious of others or believes that others are envious of him/her.
- Shows arrogant, haughty behaviors, or attitudes.

(American Psychiatric Association, 2000)

Treatment of Narcissistic Personality Disorder
- Psychotherapy: Psychoanalytic therapy approach
- Pharmacotherapy:
  - Mood stabilizers for mood swings.
  - SSRIs for those prone to depression.

## Psychotic Prone Personality Disorders
- Borderline Personality Disorder
- Schizotypal Personality Disorder
- Paranoid Personality Disorder

## Borderline Personality Disorder
Defensive structure is delayed developmentally and includes magical thinking, preoccupation with internal fantasy worlds, and tendencies to act impulsively or out of rage. When pressured these individuals may experience micropsychotic episodes, which may last from minutes to a few hours. The individual BORDERS between neurotic and psychotic, and copes with and experiences life as if there were no inner self. He feels empty and hollow unless filled with the presence of others. He experiences intense feelings of self-loathing. He is highly unpredictable and exhibits repetitive self-destructive acts. He may seek stimulation using drugs, sex, and eating to satisfy feelings of emptiness and to avoid painful feelings. Borderline personality disorder is most closely associated with paternal psychiatric maladjustments and sexual abuse and is more strongly related to paternal rather than maternal factors.

Prevalence
- Often co-occurs with mood disorders.
- It is distinguished from histrionic personality disorder by self-destructiveness, angry disruptions in close relationships, and chronic feelings of deep emptiness and loneliness.

Diagnostic Criteria
- A pervasive pattern of instability of interpersonal relationships, self-image, and affects, and marked impulsivity beginning by early adulthood and present in a variety of contexts, as indicated by five (or more) of the following:
  - Frantic efforts to avoid real or imagined abandonment.
  - A pattern of unstable and intense interpersonal relationships characterized by alternating between extremes of idealization and devaluation.

- Identity disturbance: markedly and persistently unstable self-image or sense of self.
- Impulsivity in at least two areas that are potentially self-damaging (e.g., spending, sex, substance abuse, reckless driving, binge eating).
- Recurrent suicidal behavior, gestures, or threats, or self-mutilating behavior.
- Affective instability due to a marked reactivity of mood (e.g., intense episodic dysphoria, irritability, or anxiety usually lasting for a few hours and only rarely more than a few days).
- Chronic feelings of emptiness.
- Inappropriate, intense anger or difficulty controlling anger (e.g., frequent displays of temper, constant anger, recurrent physical fights).
- Transient, stress-related paranoid ideation or severe dissociative symptoms.

(American Psychiatric Association, 2000).

Treatment of Borderline Personality Disorder:
- Psychotherapy:
  - Treatment of choice is Dialectical Behavior Therapy (DBT). DBT focuses on four groups of skills:
    - Core mindfulness skills
    - Interpersonal effectiveness skills
    - Emotion modulation skills
    - Distress tolerance skills

- Pharmacotherapy:
  - Antipsychotics to control anger, hostility, and brief psychotic episodes.
  - Antidepressants to improve mood.
  - MAOIs can modulate impulsive behaviors.
  - Anticonvulsants (i.e,. Tegretol) may improve global functioning for some patients.

*Schizotypal Personality Disorder*
Symptoms include internal blandness, vivid fantasy, and psychoses. Internal world is filled with clairvoyant messages, ghost-like appearances, and magical hunches. Individuals with this disorder are sensitive to rejection and they retreat from life. They want to make contact, but are unable to know how to do it.

Prevalence
- It is associated with paternal emotional abuse and paternal psychological maladjustment.
- It occurs in 3% of the general population.
- It has a relatively stable course, with only a small group going on to develop schizophrenia or another psychotic disorder.
- It is more prevalent among the first-degree biological relatives of individuals with schizophrenia.

Diagnostic Criteria
- *Criterion A:* A pervasive pattern of social and interpersonal deficits marked by acute discomfort with, and decreased capacity for, close relationships as well as by

cognitive or perceptual distortions and eccentricities of behavior, beginning by early adulthood and present in a variety of contexts, as indicated by five (or more) of the following:

- Ideas of reference (excluding delusions of reference).
- Odd beliefs or magical thinking that influences behavior and is inconsistent with subcultural norms (e.g., superstitiousness, belief in clairvoyance, telepathy, or "sixth sense"; in children and adolescents, bizarre fantasies or preoccupation).
- Unusual perceptual experiences, including bodily illusions.
- Odd thinking and speech (e.g., vague, circumstantial, metaphorical, over-elaborate, or stereotyped).
- Suspiciousness or paranoid ideation.
- Inappropriate or constricted affect.
- Behavior or appearance that is odd, eccentric, or peculiar.
- Lack of close friends or confidants other than first-degree relatives.
- Excessive social anxiety that does not diminish with familiarity and tends to be associated with paranoid fears rather than negative judgments of self.
- *Criterion B:* Does not occur exclusively during the course of schizophrenia, a mood disorder with psychotic features, another psychotic disorder, or a pervasive developmental disorder.

(American Psychiatric Association, 2000)

Differential Diagnoses
- 30–50% have concurrent diagnoses of major depressive disorder when admitted to a clinical setting.
- There is considerable co-occurrence with schizoid, paranoid, avoidant, and borderline personality disorder.

Treatment of Schizotypal Personality Disorder
- Psychotherapy
- Pharmacotherapy: Antipsychotics to deal with ideas of reference, illusions, and other psychotic symptoms.

## Paranoid Personality Disorder

Individuals have a deep rooted sense of inferiority, a thick coat of worrying, and see the world as a hostile environment. They see all new faces as potential enemies rather than as potential friends. They may appear "cold" and lacking of tender feelings. They are often hostile, stubborn, and have sarcastic expressions. They have a labile range of affect and are predisposed to more severe disorders on Axis I (e.g., paranoid disorder).

Prevalence
- 0.5–2.5% in the general population.
- 10–30% among those in inpatient psychiatric settings.
- 2–10% among those in outpatient mental health clinics.
- There is a familial pattern in relatives with chronic schizophrenia and a more specific familial relationship with delusional disorder, persecutory type.

Diagnostic Criteria

- A pervasive suspiciousness and distrust of others such that their motives are interpreted as malevolent, beginning by early adulthood and present in a variety of contexts, as indicated by four (or more) of the following:

  - Suspects, without sufficient basis, that others are exploiting, harming, or deceiving him/her.

  - Is preoccupied with unjustified doubts about the loyalty or trustworthiness of friends or associates.

  - Is reluctant to confide in others because of unwarranted fear that the information will be used maliciously against him or her.

  - Reads hidden demeaning or threatening meanings into benign remarks or events.

  - Persistently bears grudges (e.g., is unforgiving of insults, injuries or slights).

  - Perceives attacks on his/her character or reputation that are not apparent to others and is quick to react angrily or to counterattack.

  - Has recurrent suspicions, without justification, regarding fidelity of spouse or sexual partner.

(American Psychiatric Association, 2000)

The personality disorder must have been present before the onset of psychotic symptoms and must persist when the psychotic symptoms are in remission. Paranoid personality disorder needs to be distinguished from personality change due to a general medical condition.

Differential Diagnoses
- Delusional disorder, persecutory type.
- Schizophrenia, paranoid type.
- Mood disorder with psychotic features.

Treatment of Paranoid Personality Disorder
- Psychotherapy is the treatment of choice.
- Pharmacotherapy.
- Antipsychotics are useful in dealing with agitation and anxiety.

Personality Disorder, NOS
This category is for disorders of personality functioning that do not meet the criteria for any specific personality disorder. Features from more than one personality disorder may cause significant distress or impairment in one or more important areas of functioning (e.g., social, or occupational).

## Substance-Related Disorders and Treatment

Chemical dependency is a disease affecting an individual's mind-body-spirit, while having a significant impact upon the individual's social being and system. The disease is developed and manifested by genetic, biological, psychosocial, and environmental factors. The disease affects not only the individual, but also significant other(s), family members, and others involved (e.g., coworkers), physically, spiritually, psychologically, and socially.

## Definitions

*Addiction:* A substitute satisfaction for essential unmet needs. Dependency upon a substance, drug, or object characterized by chronic, obsessive thoughts about the substance, drug, or object and accompanying psychological and/or physiological cravings and urges for and compulsive behavior utilized in obtaining the substance, drug or object.

*Craving:* An intense psychological desire for a substance

*Tolerance:* Repeated administration of a drug results in a need for larger doses of the drug to achieve the same effect or less effect with the same dose.

*Cross-tolerance:* A client who is tolerant to a drug/substance is also physically/psychologically addicted to other drugs within a similar class. An example is when a client is psychologically and/or physiologically addicted to alcohol he or she would also be addicted to other CNS depressants such as benzodiazepines (e.g., Ativan or Klonopin).

*Drug/Substance Abuse:* Use of a substance that is not culturally acceptable. There is impairment in roles, family, occupation, legal, social, interpersonal, or medical complications as a result of usage.

*Drug/Substance Dependence:* Continuing usage of a substance despite negative consequences (e.g., DUI, loss of family, job, home). Loss of control and time spent consuming the substance(s) continue despite physical/psychological problems

*Psychological Dependence:* An internal belief that one needs the drug/substance in order to survive.

*Physiological Dependence:* Occurs when the body displays symptoms of withdrawal when the individual abstains from the drug/substance. Addiction equals dependence. An individual can be psychologically dependent on a substance(s), but not physiologically dependent. When an individual is physiologically dependent on a drug/substance, there is also psychological dependency.

*Withdrawal:* A substance-specific syndrome when the drug(s) is stopped or decreased.

*Detoxification:* Use of a drug from the same substance classification to treat objective withdrawal signs. (e.g., use of a CNS depressant such as Librium or Valium to treat withdrawal symptoms from alcohol).

*Intoxication:* A specific set of substance-specific symptoms displayed after heavy usage of a drug/substance. Remember, intoxication contains the word "toxic." At very high levels of the substance/drug it can be lethal.

*Relapse:* Recurrence of the disease state after a period of abstinence.

*Co-morbidity:* The presence of one or more additional psychiatric diagnoses in a individual who has a diagnosis of an alcohol-related disorder.

*Dual Diagnosis:* Presence of a psychiatric diagnosis in a individual who has a diagnosis of a substance-related disorder.

## Criteria for Diagnosis

The DSM-IV-TR provides criteria for the diagnosis of substance abuse, dependence, and intoxication. The nurse is an essential health care team member that can assist in gathering vital information that may substantiate a diagnosis of substance abuse, dependence, and/or intoxication.

*Substance abuse,* per DSM-IV-TR, is a maladaptive substance use pattern causing clinically significant distress or impairment, as evidenced by one or more of the following within a 12-month period:

- Persistent substance abuse with the outcome of failure in fulfilling major role responsibilities at home, work, or school.
- Persistent substance use in situations in which it is physically dangerous.
- Persistent legal problems related to substance use.
- Substance use continues regardless of continuous social and interpersonal problems created or exacerbated by the substance effects.

*Substance intoxication,* per DSM IV TR, is:
- A substance-specific syndrome caused by recent ingestion of a mood-altering substance.
- Maladaptive psychological and behavioral changes experienced are caused by substances that have an effect on the central nervous system which develop during or shortly after use of the substance.
- Symptoms that are not caused by a general medical condition or by another mental disorder.

*Substance withdrawal,* per DSM IV TR is:
- A substance-specific syndrome that develops due to the reduction of or cessation of heavy and prolonged substance use.
- Evidenced by clinically significant impairment or distress in occupational, social, or other significant areas of functioning caused by the substance-specific syndrome.
- Not caused by a general medical condition or other mental disorder.

The following test can be used to assist in the diagnosis of substance/chemical abuse and addiction.

Cage Questionnaire
There are four questions associated with this tool that can be used to assess the client's drinking habits and patterns. These questions include:

- Have you ever felt you should **C**ut down on your alcohol intake?
- Have individuals **A**nnoyed you by criticizing your alcohol intake?
- Have you ever felt **G**uilty about your alcohol intake?
- Have you ever needed alcohol for an **E**ye-opener (morning consumption)?

An affirmative answer to two or more of these questions indicates probable alcoholism. Any single affirmative answer requires further nursing assessment of the client's alcohol consumption (Ewing, 1984).

## Withdrawal from Substances

*Withdrawal* is defined as the symptoms seen when a mood-altering substance is discontinued. Withdrawal is largely dependent upon the half-life of the substance. It is important to note the duration, amount, date, time of last usage of the substance along with the half-life of the substance to calculate the potential for withdrawal.

Withdrawal symptoms will occur if the individual is physiologically dependent upon the substance. Withdrawal will begin anywhere between the numbers indicated as the half-life of the drug. This means that if the half-life of Ativan is 10–20 hours, withdrawal will begin anywhere between 10 and 20 hours after the last use of the substance.

To find out how long one would need to observe someone for withdrawal symptoms, multiply the half-life of the drug/substance by five (e.g., Ativan withdrawal can occur up to 100 hours after the last use; 20 x 5 = 100). Example: The half-life of Valium is 90–200 hours. 90 x 5 = 450 hours, 200 x 5 =1000 hours; therefore, a patient would need to be observed for Valium withdrawal symptoms from 90 up to 1000 hours. If no withdrawal symptoms are seen within that period, the nurse would know that the patient would no longer be at risk for benzodiazepine withdrawal.

Alcohol withdrawal will occur anywhere between 8 and 12 hours. Some articles report alcohol withdrawal as early as 4 hours and it may continue up to 5 days. Treatment of the withdrawal syndrome depends upon the type of drug taken. Withdrawal needs to be managed medically and slowly titrated.

Generally titration is by the same drug or one within the same drug category and is done by replacing with an alternate sedative/hypnotic (e.g., Valium, Librium), and converting dosages to comparable amounts (e.g., reduce daily intake by 50%, titrate by 5–10% per day).

The client needs to be kept comfortable and safe during the withdrawal process to motivate him or her for recovery. A history of a seizure during withdrawal from alcohol is most likely to occur again during subsequent alcohol withdrawal if the client is not medicated to prevent the seizure. It is important to note that a mood-stabilizing anti-convulsant such as Depakote or Neurontin WILL NOT prevent a withdrawal seizure. Only phenobarbital will prevent an alcohol withdrawal-related seizure.

## Categories of Drugs/Substances

*Sedatives/Hypnotics*
This category includes:
• Alcohol

• Benzodiazepines (minor tranquilizers) – Partial List
  • Librium          • Ativan          • Xanax
  • Tanxene          • Valium          • Dalmane
  • Serax            • Restoril        • Halcion
  • Klonopin         • Limbritol

• Barbiturates (major tranquilizers) – Partial List
  • Phenobarbital    • Pentothal       • Amytal
  • Tuinal           • Butisol         • Nembutal
  • Seconal          • Fiorinal        • Brevital
  • Luminal

• Antihistamines – Partial List
  • Benadryl         • Phenergan       • Vistaril

• Sedatives – Partial List
  • Chloral Hydrate  • Equinil         • Valmid
  • Bromides         • Parest          • Noctec
  • Somnos           • Perichlor       • Betachlor
  • Sopar            • Chloretone      • Paraldehyde

*Signs of intoxication* from these substances, primarily due to CNS depression, include: decreased pulse, respiration and blood pressure, dry and flushed skin, drowsiness, slurred speech, GI tract slowing, slowed thought processes, and slowed reflexes.

*Signs of withdrawal* from these substances, primarily due to CNS hyperactivity, include: elevated pulse, respiration, and blood pressure, diaphoresis, pallor, insomnia, anorexia, anxiety, restlessness, GI tract hyperactivity, hyperactive thought processes, hyperreflexia, nausea, vomiting, and tremors.

## Medical Consequences of Sedative/Hypnotic Usage

### Alcohol

*Brain Atrophy: Wernicke-Korsakoff's Syndrome:* This is one of the most commonly found conditions in the chronic alcoholic. It occurs primarily from a deficiency in thiamine (Vitamin B-1). Thiamine is essential for the functioning of nerve tissues, such as the peripheral nerves and the brain. With prolonged alcohol use, there is insufficient dietary intake and poor absorption of thiamine. Symptoms include sudden marked confusion, unsteady gait, double vision, and uncoordinated movement. The condition requires prompt treatment with large amounts of thiamine within the first few hours to first few days.

If thiamine is not given within this time period, death may result or the client will develop the Korsakoff's part of the condition. Symptoms of the Korsakoff's portion of the illness include: marked impairment of memory, disorientation to person, place, date, and time, an inability to retain memory of ongoing events, and short-term memory loss. The client will most likely have peripheral neuropathy. The outlook once Korsakoff's syndrome has been established is poor.

*Chronic subdural hematoma* may develop due to the frequent falls to which the alcoholic individual is prone. The client may have fallen days to weeks prior to presenting for treatment. Symptoms may include dizziness, headaches, convulsions, and paralysis on one side of the body. The pupil of the eye may be dilated on the side of the hematoma. Symptoms resembling psychiatric disorders may also result, such as periods of confusion, anxiety, depression, odd behavior, and suspiciousness. Brain cells are destroyed by alcohol use and once destroyed they cannot be rejuvenated.

*Gastritis* can develop because alcohol causes an increase in production of stomach acid. Symptoms include upper abdominal pain, indigestion, nausea, and/or decreased appetite. Infrequently, vomiting of blood may result due to the erosions of the stomach lining (e.g., Mallory-Weiss tear).

*Pancreatitis,* an inflammation of the pancreas, has symptoms of acute abdominal pain, nausea, and vomiting.

*Diarrhea* can result as alcohol causes the retention of water and salt in the intestine and encourages strong movements within the intestine.

*Fatty Liver:* The liver is the detoxification center of the body and breaks down and disposes of alcohol. The liver is able to dispose of only a certain amount of alcohol in a given time period. The liver becomes heavy with fat that is accumulated. Symptoms include upper abdominal tenderness and pain. Symptoms may be minimal or absent.

*Alcoholic Hepatitis:* Inflammation of the liver due to the toxic effects of alcohol upon the liver; middle stage between fatty liver and liver cirrhosis. Symptoms may include "flu-like" symptoms, tenderness over the enlarged liver, right upper abdominal pain, fever, chills, nausea, vomiting, and jaundice.

*Ascites:* fluid accumulation in the abdominal cavity.

*Alcoholic cirrhosis of the liver* involves severe damage to the liver; it develops scar tissue and the liver becomes "inactive." The liver will atrophy and may become rock hard or nodular. Diagnosis generally occurs in middle-aged alcoholics and occurs when the client experiences a state of confusion. Symptoms include jaundice and palmar erythema (a reddening of the palms of the hands).

*Espophageal varices* are pockets of blood that accumulate in the varicose veins in the esophagus. Esophageal bleeds seen in the ER are often caused by chronic alcoholism.

*Portal hypertension* occurs when blood is blocked in the liver, cannot flow freely through the liver, and requires finding another route to the heart. This causes undue pressure on the vein systems that are already vulnerable—the esophagus and the stomach. Portal hypertension is NOT associated with high blood pressure.

*Cardiac arrhythmias* may result from consumption of small to moderate amounts of alcohol. Drinking alcohol along with caffeinated beverages will predispose an individual to developing an arrhythmia.

*Coronary artery disease* is the narrowing of the blood vessels due to accumulation of fatty substances.

*Alcoholic cardiomyopathy* is heart muscle damage. The individual complains of shortness of breath, peripheral edema, decreased tissue perfusion to the nail beds, fatigue, and palpitations.

*Peripheral neuropathy* occurs from a decrease of thiamine in the nerves in the arms and legs of the individual. Symptoms commonly associated with peripheral neuropathy include a prickling, tingling or burning sensation in the fingers and feet.

*Diminished sexual desire and potency* is a frequent complaint by chronic alcoholics.

*Gynecomastia* (enlargement of the breast area) can result in men because alcohol increases the mount of estrogen in the male. Atrophy of the testicles may also result. An impairment in erection and/or ejaculation may also be experienced. Physical arousal in the woman may be impaired with prolonged alcohol use.

*Fetal alcohol syndrome* is associated with excessive maternal alcohol consumption during pregnancy, which can cause one or more of the following defects:
• small head
• low birth weight
• short body length
• slow growth after birth
• narrowed eye slits
• underdeveloped facial structure
• flattened cheek bones
• abnormally thin upper lip
• mental retardation
• delayed development

*Sleep Disturbances:* During the sobering-up period, there is an increase in rapid eye movements; the client may complain of restlessness during sleep, vivid dreams, and/or nightmares. During the weeks to months after alcohol cessation, sleep may be restless, and there can be frequent yet unremembered awakenings.

## Other Sedative/Hypnotics

Intentional or unintentional overdoses; seizures; restlessness, delirium, muscle spasms, convulsions, and death. Dangers of IV barbiturate use include: risk of transmission of HIV, cellulitis, vascular complications from accidental injection into an artery, infections, and allergic reactions.

## Treatment of Withdrawal from Sedative Hypnotics

*Nursing Intervention*

- Assess vital signs every 2–4 hours and medicate per institution protocol.
- Administer benzodiazepine (the same one utilized by client or another similar benzodiazepine) per detox protocol, and taper dosages per protocol.
- It is imperative the client receive his/her scheduled dosages and not miss or skip dosages because of the potential for seizure, especially with benzodiazepine dependency.
- Educate client regarding the withdrawal process and that client will be kept safe.
- Educate client to not participate in strenuous exercise until post-withdrawal monitoring is complete.
- Administer 100 mg thiamine by mouth three times per day for alcohol withdrawal to treat peripheral neuropathy. May also administer IM.
- Instruct client to increase fluid intake.
- Provide comfort measures for reducing nausea/vomiting, such as applying cool, moist cloth to forehead or back of neck and cool, clear liquids.
- Assist client with hygiene/grooming as needed.
- Provide comfort measures for client to reduce distress.
- Teach deep breathing techniques
- Have client listen to soothing music
- Instruct client detoxing from benzodiazepines to avoid strenuous exercise, because benzodiazepines are stored in fat cells and exercise would cause the benzodiazepine to be released more quickly—withdrawal symptoms could worsen and possibly lead to seizure activity.
- Instruct client to be honest regarding symptoms experienced so that the safest/best nursing care can be provided.

## Opioid Type (Narcotics)

Substances include:

- Morphine
- Dilaudid
- Methadone
- Darvocet
- Lomotil
- Codeine
- Hycodan
- Demerol
- Stadol
- Heroin
- Percodan
- Darvon
- Talwin

## Medical Consequences of Opiate Abuse

One of the most common and serious adverse effects associated with the use of opioids is the potential risk of transmission of HIV and hepatitis through the use of contaminated needles by more than one individual. Other adverse effects include abscesses. Death from an overdose of an opiate is generally due to respiratory arrest from the respiratory depressant effects of the drug.

*Opiate intoxication* can be exhibited by analgesia, apathy, drowsiness, drooling, euphoria, flushed skin, itching, nodding, peripheral vasodilation, slowed speech, spontaneous orgasm, and respiratory depression.

*Opiate withdrawal* can be exhibited by abdominal spasms, anorexia, chills, dehydration, depression, diarrhea, elevated temperature and pulse, flushed skin, gooseflesh, irritability, lacrimation, muscle cramps, rhinorrhea, sneezing, vomiting, weight loss, and yawning.

*Opiate overdose* is exhibited by shallow breathing, tachycardia, hypotension, depressed levels of consciousness, clammy skin, convulsions, papillary dilation, unconsciousness, coma, and death.

The antidote for opioid (narcotic) overdose is Narcan.

## Nursing Interventions for Opiate Withdrawal

- Withdrawal symptoms generally subside within 5–7 days. However, prodromal symptoms of insomnia, drug craving, anhedonia, and dysphoria can last from a period of weeks to months.
- Nursing interventions for withdrawal management focus on alleviation of discomfort and symptom management.
- Monitor vital signs and administer clonidine (Catapres), an opioid antagonist, transdermally and orally to assist in blocking opioid receptor sites and to prevent and/or alleviate withdrawal symptoms.
- Provide soothing measures for client based on symptoms; for example, warm blankets to assist in alleviating chills, non-steroidal anti-inflammatory medication prn for comfort, provide warm whirlpool baths as available.
- Provide client with sleep hygiene measures
  - Avoid extremes of temperature, loud noises, illuminated clocks
  - Provide only a "mild" nightlight, if necessary
  - Provide hs (before bedtime) snack
  - Listen to relaxation tapes
  - Avoid daytime naps
  - Discontinue CNS-acting drugs
- Provide anti-diarrheal medication if needed.
- Provide continual reassurance to client as he or she craves the opiate.
- Provide adequate hydration.
- Offer diversional activities to client.
- Provide interventions to alleviate nausea and vomiting.
- Place a cool cloth on forehead, back of neck.
- Offer carbonated beverages.
- Teach deep breathing techniques.

- Provide a calm environment with supportive care.
- Teach client medical consequences of opiate abuse.

- Stimulants – Partial List
  - Cocaine
  - Amphetamines
    - Dexedrine
    - Methamphetamine
    - Cylert
    - Ritalin
  - Adderall
  - Crank
  - Crystal methamphetamine
  - Speed
  - D-Amphetamine
  - Benzedrine
  - Melfiat
  - Phendiet
  - Preludin
  - Ionamin
  - Tepanil
  - Methadrine
  - Didrex
  - Paredrine

Medical Consequences of Amphetamines:
- HIV, hepatitis, and development of lung abscesses, and endocarditis. Amphetamines are often used to enhance sexual experiences; however, long-term use and high doses are associated with impotence and other sexual dysfunctions.

*Signs of psychostimulant intoxication* can include a sense of increased alertness, anxiety, decreased appetite, delayed orgasm, drowsiness in chronic users, elevated mood, enhanced physical strength and mental capacity, irritability, suspiciousness, psychosis, hallucinations, hypertension, elevated pulse, preoccupation, diarrhea, decreased skin temperature, repressed stomach contractions, and sleep disturbances.

*Signs of withdrawal from psychostimulants* can include agitation, cravings, decreased concentration, dullness, drowsiness, GI disturbances, labile emotions, decreased psychomotor performance, fatigue, depression, and prolonged sleep. Seizures may occur from IV cocaine withdrawal.

*Signs of overdose of psychostimulants* include arrhythmias, assaultiveness, chills, convulsions, psychosis, hallucinations, coma, diarrhea, flushing, confusion, restlessness, respiratory depression, sweating, tremors, labile blood pressure, circulatory collapse, and respiratory collapse.

## Management of Withdrawal from Psychostimulants
- Withdrawal symptoms generally subside over 2–4 days after drug abstinence.
- There is no specific treatment for stimulant withdrawal.
- Symptom management.
- Cocaine cravings usually rapidly diminish when the individual is unable to get the drug and no longer is exposed to the stimuli in the environment associated with cocaine use.
- Cocaine abusers commonly take alcohol, marijuana, or heroin with cocaine to reduce the irritability caused by high-dose stimulant abuse, thus the withdrawal may be in response to the combination of drugs.

## Hallucinogens
Drugs include:

- LSD
- STP
- Peyote
- Psilocybin
- Hashoil
- Ecstasy

- PCP
- Mescaline
- Psilocin
- Hashish
- MDMA

*Medical Consequences of Hallucinogen Abuse*

The effects are unique to each individual. Mild or severe depression, convulsions, flashbacks can occur at anytime. Death can occur from toxic drug levels, suicide, or driving under the influence.

*Signs of Intoxication:* Unpredictable alterations in thought, mood, perceptions; enhanced self-awareness; heightened sensitivity to faces, gestures, feelings are magnified; heightened body awareness; distortions of all senses occurring from excitement to terror. There is a combination of sensory experiences—what is seen is also heard. Episodes can last from minutes to days and their effects can last from hours to weeks.

Other signs may include anorexia, anxiety, dizziness, hallucinations, hyperthermia, hypertension, nausea, paresthesia, dilated pupils, suspiciousness, tachycardia, nausea, vomiting, tremor.

*Signs of overdose* include delirium, grand mal seizures, hyperthermia, paresthesia, psychosis, tremor, tachycardia, hypertension, abdominal cramps, and dilated pupils.

*Withdrawal from hallucinogens* is something not much is known about.

## Cannabis (Marijuana)
Marijuana and hashish (smoked) and tetrahydrocannabinol (oral) are included in this drug class. Cannabis is the most commonly used illicit substance in the U.S.

*Medical Consequences of Marijuana Abuse*

Many reports indicate the long-term use of cannabis is associated with cerebral atrophy, susceptibility to seizures, birth defects, chromosomal damage, alterations in concentrations of testosterone, disruption in the menstrual cycle, and an impaired immune system.

*Signs of Intoxication* include euphoria, relaxed inhibitions, impaired memory and attention, increased appetite. Motor skills are impaired. Cannabis is often used with alcohol (depressant) or stimulants such as cocaine, and nicotine. Cannabis intoxication generally heightens the user's sensitivity to external stimuli, reveals new details, will slow down the appreciation of time, and can make colors seem richer and brighter. Urine drug tests may be positive for cannabis for up to 7–10 days. In clients with very heavy use of cannabis, their urine may be positive for up to 2–4 weeks.

According to the American Psychiatric Association (2000), Cannabis intoxication is noted by:
- Recent ingestion of cannabis.

- Psychological and behavioral changes of clinical significance (e.g., euphoria, sensation of slowed time, impaired judgment) that develop during or shortly after use of cannabis.

- Two (or more) of the following symptoms develop within 2 hours after cannabis use:
  - conjunctival injection
  - increased appetite
  - dry mouth
  - tachycardia
- The symptoms are not caused by a general medical condition or by another mental illness.

*Signs of withdrawal* include anxiety, decreased appetite, hyperactivity, and insomnia.

*Signs of a toxic reaction* include fatigue, panic reactions, paranoid ideation, and psychosis.

## Other Drugs

*Phencyclidine*

Drug names: crystal, PCP, angel dust, rocket fuel, dust, peace pill.

*Signs of Intoxication* include agitation, floating sensation, lethargy, increased blood pressure, slowed reflexes, altered body image, altered perceptions of time and space, catatonic immobility, bizarre behavior, stupor, violent behavior. Symptoms last from 30 minutes to 6 hours.

*Major symptoms/patterns* are seen with this drug and are possibly dose related:

- Acute brain syndrome: disorientation, confusion, loss of recent memory, labile, inappropriate behavior, violence.
- Catatonic syndrome: mutism, negativism, posturing, possible violence, rigidity, stupor.
- Coma: mild, moderate, or severe.
- Toxic Psychosis: the patient may experience delusions/hallucinations (e.g., visual/auditory, often brightly colored lights, bizarre behavior). The onset of these symptoms may not be exhibited for up to 7 days after the ingestion of PCP; duration is 1–30 days, the average is 3–4 days.

*Dual Diagnoses and Co-Morbid Conditions.* Co-morbidity is the presence of an additional psychiatric diagnosis in an individual with a diagnosis of a substance-related disorder. This is often referred to as dual diagnosis. Some of the most common psychiatric diagnoses accompanying substance-related disorders are listed below:

- Polysubstance abuse
- Antisocial personality disorder
- Bipolar illnesses
- Major depressive disorder
- Cyclothymic disorder
- Anxiety disorders
- Posttraumatic stress disorder

*Relapse Prevention.* Relapse is a term used to describe when a individual begins to behave in a dysfunctional/unhelpful manner after a period of abstinence, recovery, or sobriety. Relapse occurs long before the actual "slip" of chemical use, or the first drink or drug use. It is a period of time leading to a relapse. Since the psychosocial aspect of caring for clients is part of the nursing role, assisting the client in identifying relapse triggers is important. Encouraging the client to enter therapy can also be extremely important.

Other treatment issues to be explored and addressed in therapy with the chemically dependent client include:

- Assessment for and treatment of co-morbid psychiatric illnesses.
- Participation in a 12-step recovery program, e.g., Alcoholics Anonymous, Narcotics Anonymous.
- Spirituality.
- Anger management.
- Stress management, anxiety reduction.
- Attachment/avoidance issues.
- Reality orientation.

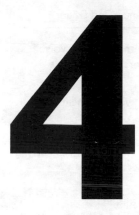

# Treatment Modalities

## Biological Therapies: Psychopharmacology

### Neuroanatomy and Physiology
*Overall Brain Structure*

The brain consists of three components:
- Cerebrum
- Brain stem
- Cerebellum

*Cerebrum*
The cerebrum consists of two hemispheres: the right and the left. The hemispheres can be further divided into four major lobes: frontal, temporal, parietal, and occipital.

*Frontal lobe:* high level cognitive functioning occurs in this area, such as executive control, abstraction, concentration, reasoning, complex decision-making. Other functions include:
- Emotions.
- Storage of information (memory).
- Control of voluntary eye movements.
- Influence of somatic motor control of activities such as respiration, GI activity, and blood pressure.
- Motor control of speech in the dominant hemisphere (usually the left hemisphere).

Lesions in this area can create loss of ability to integrate both internal and external environmental clues and to pursue any goal-directed behaviors

*Parietal lobe:* Sensory input is interpreted to define size, shape, weight, and consistency.
- Sensation is localized and modalities of touch, pressure, and position are identified.
- Individual's awareness of parts of the body is the function of the parietal lobe.
- The dominant parietal lobe is involved in ideomotor praxis (motor movement) and the nondominant parietal lobe is involved in processing visual-spatial orientation.

*Temporal lobe:* The primary auditory receptive areas are located in this area (Wernicke's area).
- This area is usually largest in the dominant hemisphere. If damage occurs to the Wernicke's area, words are heard, but the individual is unable to interpret the meaning.

- The interpretive area is located in the temporal lobe. Memory that would involve more than one sensory modality, such as artwork, music, conversations, or past experiences, is stored in this area.

*Occipital lobe:* Visual perception, reflexes, and involuntary smooth eye movement.

The cerebrum also includes the basal ganglia, thalamus, hypothalamus, and limbic system.

*Basal Ganglia:* A group of deep nuclei within the cerebral hemisphere involved in the feedback regulation of voluntary and involuntary movement.
- It mediates motor activity: EPS (extrapyramidal symptoms).
- Has a role in the expression and regulation of emotion and cognition.
- Huntington chorea is caused by atrophy of the caudate nucleus. Symptoms include dementia and involuntary choreiform movements.

*Thalamus:* Deep brain structure having many nuclei. Function is to perceive and relay motor and sensory information. The thalamus is a relay station.

*Hypothalamus:* Located beneath the thalamus and on either side of the third ventricle, involved in the regulation of:
- sleep
- appetite
- sexual activity
- hormonal regulation
- autonomic functioning
- memory and learning
- temperature control, BP, and heart rate

Nerves in the hypothalamus relay messages from the autonomic nervous system (ANS) and command the body through those nerves and the pituitary.

*Limbic System:* A group of subcortical nuclei involved in the emotions of fear, sexual drive, hunger, sleep, and short-term memory. Included within the limbic system are the amygdala, hippocampus, septum, and parts of the cortex. These brain structures experience and regulate emotions, regulate memory, and are involved in learning (hippocampus and amygdala) and integration of sensory data from the environment. Lesions in the amygdala lead to fearfulness, suspiciousness, and paranoia.

*Hippocampus:* A single midline structure located at the roof of the third ventricle whose major function is secretion of melatonin, which is involved in the sleep-wake cycle.

The *corpus callosum* connects cerebral hemispheres to each other. The corpus callosum CALLS the two cerebral hemispheres together.

## Brain Stem

The brain stem consists of the midbrain, pons, and medulla.

*Midbrain:* Involved in auditory and visual reflexes, channels the reticular activating system (RAS) up to the thalamus.

*Pons:* Involved with respiratory function, channels RAS from medulla to midbrain.

*Medulla oblongata:* A brainstem organ responsible for the basic functions of regulating blood pressure, respiration, sleep, and consciousness. The RAS begins here.

The *brain stem* contains the centers for sneezing, coughing, hiccupping, vomiting, sucking, and swallowing.

*Cerebellum*
The function of the cerebellum is to coordinate voluntary movement, maintain trunk stability, and maintain equilibrium.

## Neurotransmitters
Three major types of neurotransmitters are:
* biogenic amines (monoamines)
  * histamine
  * acetylcholine
  * serotonin (5HT-2)
  * dopamine (DA)
  * norepinephrine (NE)
  * epinephrine (E)
  * catecholamines
* amino acids
* peptides

*Action*
*Uptake:* major factor in termination of action.
*Reuptake:* means recycled.

## Serotonin (5HT-2) ↑→ *help depression*
*Synthesis*: Precursor is tryptophan. Must be taken up into the brain; plasma tryptophan arises primarily from diet. Foods which are known to assist in producing tryptophan and ultimately serotonin include: papaya, pineapple, pumpkin, sunflower seeds, turkey, red plums, blue red plums, tomatoes, avocados, eggplant, and passion fruit. ? milk

Drugs that work by keeping more serotonin available in the synapses (site of action) are called specific serotonin reuptake inhibitors (SSRIs), such as fluoxetine (Prozac), paroxetine (Paxil), and sertraline (Zoloft). Note: SSRIs could be called SSUIs since they are actually selective serotonin-uptake inhibitors, e.g., keeping more serotonin available in the synapses.

*Neuronal structure includes:* cell body, nerve fibers, and dendrites.

## General Principles of Psychopharmacology
*Factors Affecting Drug Therapy*

Hepatic and renal functioning play the major roles in the metabolism of drugs. Drugs are either fat or water-soluble. The liver is the main center of metabolism for fat-soluble medications. Water-soluble drugs are easily excreted via the urine. Psychoactive drugs are usually fat-soluble.

The biological half-life of drugs (T-1/2) is the amount of time it takes for the body to eliminate one-half of the drug molecules from the blood stream.

The aging process affects the metabolism of medications in several ways. Dosages for the older adult need careful consideration. With aging, functional changes occur in many of the systems that control the drug metabolism process. Drugs have a tendency to be absorbed, distributed, metabolized, and excreted more slowly and less effectively. This results in a prolonged action of the drugs. Increased half-life may produce toxic accumulations. Cardiac output normally decreases with age. With a decrease in cardiac reserve and regional blood flow and an increase in circulation time, there is an altered absorption and distribution rate. Body fat increases the duration of activity of highly lipid-soluble drugs. Body fat increases with age, especially in females. This is another reason for an increased potential for toxicity.

## Controlled Substances Act

The Comprehensive Drug Abuse Prevention and Control Act of 1970 was designed to provide increased research into and prevention of drug abuse and drug dependence, to provide for treatment and rehabilitation of drug abusers and drug dependent individuals, and to strengthen existing law enforcement authority in the field of drug abuse. The Controlled Substances Act schedules or classifies drugs according to medical usefulness and potential for abuse.

*Schedule I.* Drugs that currently do not have accepted medical use and have a high abuse potential, e.g., heroin, marijuana, LSD.

*Schedule II.* Drugs that have a medical use but a high abuse potential with severe dependence liability, e.g., some narcotics, some barbiturates, amphetamines.

*Schedule III.* Drugs used in medical practice that have less potential for abuse than those in Schedule II and moderate dependence liability, e.g., nonbarbiturate sedatives, nonamphetamine stimulants, anabolic steroids, and certain narcotics.

*Schedule IV.* Drugs that have medical use, less potential for abuse than those in Schedule III, and limited dependence liability, e.g., anxiolytics, some sedatives, non-narcotic analgesics.

*Schedule V.* Drugs that have medical use and limited abuse potential, e.g., small amounts of narcotics, such as codeine used in antitussives or antidiarrheals.

## Factors Used in Selecting a Specific Psychotropic Medication (Nihart & Laraia, 1994, p. 27)

*Primary Considerations*
- Side effect profile of the medication
- Ease of administration, e.g., route, number of times to administer per day, need to be refrigerated
- History of past response
- Current safety/medical conditions
- Specific subtype (if applicable)

*Secondary Considerations*
- Neurotransmitter selectivity: when one medication does not work, consider a second or third-line drug
- Family history of response
- Blood level considerations
- Cost of medication

## Phases of Psychopharmacologic Management

*Initiation*
- Pharmacokinetics/pharmacodynamics
- Client education about medication and alternative treatment—informed consent
- Identification of target symptoms and rating scales
- Early medication effects
- Alternative treatments
- Development of treatment plans
- Implications of information obtained in assessment

*Stabilization*
- Continued assessment of target symptoms, e.g., rating scales, BP, lab results, individual rating scale 1–10
- Expected timing of medication effects, e.g., some therapeutic levels are seen at 3–4 weeks
- Recognition and treatment of adverse effects, e.g., especially with tardive dyskinesia, serotonin syndrome, neuroleptic malignant syndrome
- Therapeutic drug monitoring, e.g., tricyclics, lithium, depakote, neurontin
- When and how to change medication strategies
- Ongoing patient education
- Transition between treatment settings

*Maintenance (relapse of illness can occur at this point)*
- Education regarding relapse and recognition of stressors
- Monitoring efficacy, side effects and laboratory values
- Consider long-term side effect potential—address compliance issues
- When and how to discontinue medication treatment
- Patient education for relapse prevention

*Medication-Free*
- Duration of treatment for a given disorder
- Tapering methods/schedules
- Symptom recognition
- Relapse prevention

## Pharmacological Agents Used to Treat Psychiatric Disorders
*Antipsychotics*
Antipsychotic or neuroleptic medications are used to treat acute psychotic symptoms such as hallucinations, paranoia, and delusions, regardless of the cause of the psychosis. They are most often used in chronic mental illnesses such as schizophrenia. They are also used to treat agitation, nightmares, and thought disorders.

Commonly used antipsychotics, whether typical or atypical, have a variety of potencies. The standard dose of 100 mg chlorpromazine (Thorazine) is used to approximate dose equivalents of commonly used agents. As an example, a 2 mg dose of fluphenazine (Prolixin) has a therapeutic effect with an approximate equivalence of 100 mg of chlorpromazine.

*Typical Antipsychotics:* Conventional or typical antipsychotic medications were invented about 50 years ago. These drugs relieve psychotic symptoms and have allowed a multitude of patients to leave psychiatric hospitals and live in less restrictive environments in the community. These drugs, however, have limitations. They are not very effective for the full range of symptoms experienced by individuals with severe mental illnesses. Negative symptoms, such as apathy, withdrawal, and lack of emotion, and cognitive symptoms, such as comprehension, judgment, memory, and reasoning, are not improved. In fact, the cognitive symptoms are often worsened by the sedative effect of these medications. In addition, side effects are a major problem with this type of medication.

Side effects include:
- Extrapyramidal reactions
  - Dystonias: spasms in major muscle groups of eyes, neck, and back occurring suddenly.
  - Pseudoparkinsonism: cogwheel rigidity, slowness of motion, small shuffling gait, mask-like face, pill-rolling motion of the fingers.
  - Akathisia: motor restlessness.
  - Tardive dyskinesia: stereotypical involuntary movement disorder usually involving the mouth, face, neck, and upper extremities; lip smacking, tongue protrusion, chewing, grimacing, choreiform movements of limbs and trunk.
- Anticholinergic side effects: nasal congestion, dry mouth, blurred vision, constipation, urinary retention.
- Other side effects: seizures, sedation, postural hypotension, photosensitivity, weight gain, amenorrhea, decreased libido.
- Life threatening: neuroleptic malignant syndrome.

*Table 4-1. Typical Antipsychotics*

| Generic Name | Trade Name | Avg. Daily Dose | Notes/Precautions |
|---|---|---|---|
| chlorpromazine | Thorazine | 50–200 mg | |
| droperidol | Inapsine | 2.5–10 mg | IM only. Monitor patient closely for CNS depression |
| fluphenazine | Prolixin | 2–40 mg | Available in long acting IM, decanoate form. |
| haloperidol | Haldol | 2–40 mg | Available in long acting IM, decanoate form. |
| loxapine | Loxitane | 20–250 mg | |
| mesoridazine | Serentil | 75–900 mg | |
| molindone | Moban | 50–225 mg | |
| perphenazine | Trilafon | 8–64 mg | |
| thioridazine | Mellaril | 50–800 mg | |
| thiothixene | Navane | 5–60 mg | |
| trifluoperazine | Stelazine | 10–80 mg | |

*Atypical Antipsychotics:* In 1990, a new generation of antipsychotic medications was born with the invention of clozapine (Clozaril). The atypical antipsychotics not only treat the positive symptoms of psychotic illnesses but also the negative and cognitive symptoms. In addition, the side effect profile is much improved. These medications are more specific for neurotransmitter effects. The incidence of extrapyramidal reactions is greatly diminished, almost to the point that it is in placebo with some medications. The risk of tardive dyskinesia is also significantly lowered.

The lives of individuals with chronic and pervasive mental illnesses have been greatly improved with the advent of this generation of antipsychotic medications. They have their own set of side effects, however. Weight gain can be an issue with some of these medications, as can sedation. Some cause QT interval prolongation. Prolactin elevation is not seen, however, so amenorrhea, galactorrhea, and other subsequent problems are lessened.

### Table 4-2. Atypical Antipsychotics

| Generic Name | Trade Name | Avg. Daily Dose | Notes/Precautions |
|---|---|---|---|
| clozapine | Clozaril | 75–90 mg | CBC QOW, agranulocytosis risk |
| olanzapine | Zyprexa | 2.5–20 mg | Broad-spectrum psychotropic |
| quetiapine | Seroquel | 150–750 mg | |
| risperidone | Risperdal | 2–20 mg | Risk of EPSs above 8 mg |
| ziprasidone | Geodon | 20–80 mg | QT interval prolongation. Sudden death. |

*Common Side Effects:* Sedation, weight gain, hypersalivation, postural hypotension, anticholinergic side effects.
*Serious Side Effects:* Neuroleptic malignant syndrome (NMS), very low incidence. Sudden death from QT interval prolongation of ziprasidone.

### Mood Stabilizers

Multiple neurotransmitters, serotonin, norepinephrine, and gamma-amino-butyric-acid (GABA), may be involved in the process of bipolar illness. Medications that are have been used as anticonvulsants are now being used to treat mood disorders because of their effect on GABA. Olanzapine, a broad-spectrum psychotropic affecting multiple neurotransmitters, is being used successfully for bipolar illness. Some patients need both a mood stabilizer and an antidepressant if their symptoms are primarily depressive. However, a patient with bipolar illness should not be given an antidepressant alone, as it may trigger a manic episode.

### Table 4-3. Mood Stabilizers

| Generic Name | Trade Name | Average Daily Dose | Notes/Precautions |
|---|---|---|---|
| carbamazepine | Tegretol | 200–1200 mg | |
| gabapentin | Neurontin | 300–1800 mg | |
| lamotrigine | Lamictal | 100–400 mg | Stevens-Johnson syndrome |
| lithium | Eskalith | 300–1800 mg | Blood level: 0.6–1.5 meq. Toxicity. Thyroid toxicity. |
| olanzapine | Zyprexa | 5–20 mg | Indicated for bipolar illness |
| topiramate | Topamax | 50–400 mg | |
| valproic acid | Depakene | 750–3000 mg | Blood level: 50–120 mcg/m |

*Common Side Effects:* Sedation, weight gain, GI distress, tremor, thirstiness.
*Serious Side Effects:* Toxicity, hepatotoxicity.

## Antidepressants

In addition to treating clinical depression, antidepressant medications have been found to be useful for pain control, mood stabilization, bulimia nervosa, anxiety disorders, PTSD, and ADHD.

Table 4-4. Trycyclic Antidepressants

| Generic Name | Trade Name | Average Daily Dose | Notes/Precautions |
|---|---|---|---|
| amitriptyline | Elavil | 50–300 mg | |
| amoxapine | Asendin | 50–600 mg | |
| desipramine | Norpramin | 50–300 mg | |
| imipramine | Tofranil | 50–300 mg | |
| nortriptyline | Pamelor | 50–150 mg | |

Common Side Effects: Dry mouth, orthostatic hypotension, blurred vision, constipation, urinary retention, sedation.
Serious Side Effects: Cardiac toxicity, overdose.

## Monoamine Oxidase Inhibitors

A low tyramine diet is necessary when patients are treated with MAOIs. Foods containing tryptophan or tyramine, aged cheeses, red wine, soy sauce, salami, bananas, cannot be used. Hypertensive crisis, including elevated BP, headache, nausea, vomiting, sweating, and photophobia can occur if the diet is not complied with. These medications are used second or third line in the fight against depression.

Table 4-5. MAOIs

| Generic Name | Trade Name | Average Daily Dose | Notes/Precautions |
|---|---|---|---|
| isocarboxazid | Marplan | 30–70 mg | |
| phenelzine | Nardil | 45–90 mg | |
| tranylcypromine | Parnate | 20–60 mg | |

Common Side Effects: Dry mouth, blurred vision, constipation, insomnia, orthostatic hypotension.
Serious Side Effects: hypertensive crisis.

Table 4-6. Selective Serontonin Reuptake Inhibitors

| Generic Name | Trade Name | Average Daily Dose | Notes/Precautions |
|---|---|---|---|
| citalopram | Celexa | 20-60 mg | 36 hour half-life |
| escitalopram | Lexapro | 10-20 mg | 25 hour half-life |
| fluoxetine | Prozac | 10-80 mg | 36 hour half-life |
| fluvoxamine | Luvox | 100-300 mg | 14 hour half-life |
| paroxetine | Paxil | 20-60 mg | 21 hour half-life |
| sertraline | Zoloft | 50-200 mg | 26 hour half-life |

Common Side Effects: Nausea, diarrhea, sexual dysfunction, nervousness, somnolence, dry mouth.
Serious Side Effects: SSRI discontinuation syndrome with shorter half-life meds: vertigo, ataxia, nausea, parasthesia, agitation.

## Table 4-7. Other Antidepressants

| Generic Name | Trade Name | Average Daily Dose | Notes/Precautions |
|---|---|---|---|
| bupropion | Wellbutrin | 50–600 mg | dopamine reuptake inhibitor, lowers seizure threshold |
| mirtazapine | Remeron | 15–45 mg | *fever dis.* |
| nefazodone | Serzone | 300–600 mg | SNRI, contraindicated in patients with liver disease |
| trazodone | Desyrel | 400–600 mg | SNRI |
| venlafaxine | Effexor | 75–375 mg | SNRI, can cause or exacerbate hypertension |

*SNRI = Serotonin-norepinephrine reuptake inhibitor

### Anxiolytics (Antianxiety Agents)

Antianxiety agents have multiple uses: anxiety, OCD, PTSD, alcohol withdrawal, muscle spasms, and insomnia.

## Table 4-8. Antianxiety Agents

| Generic Name | Trade Name | Average Daily Dose | Notes/Precautions |
|---|---|---|---|
| alprazolam | Xanax | 2–8 mg | |
| buspirone | BuSpar | 20–30 mg | |
| chlordiazepoxide | Librium | 10–50 mg | |
| clonazepam | Klonopin | 0.5–1.5 mg | |
| diazepam | Valium | 5–30 mg | |
| lorazepam | Ativan | 2–6 mg | |
| meprobamate | Meprospan | 200–800 mg | |
| oxazepam | Serax | 10–60 mg | |

*Common Side Effects:* Sedation, confusion, tolerance.
*Serious Side Effects:* Addiction, dependence.

### Sedatives/Hypnotics

Common uses of sedatives/hypnotics include insomnia, pre-operative sedation, and agitation.

## Table 4-9. Sedatives/Hynotics

| Generic Name | Trade Name | Average Daily Dose | Notes/Precautions |
|---|---|---|---|
| chloral hydrate | Noctec | 500–1000 mg | |
| eszopiclone | Lunesta | 1-3 mg | |
| flurazepam | Dalmane | 15–30 mg | |
| pentobarbital | Nembutal | 100–200 mg | |
| temazepam | Restoril | 7.5–30 mg | |
| zaleplon | Sonata | 5–10 mg | |
| zolpidem | Ambien | 5–10 mg | |

*Common Side Effects:* sedation, tolerance.
*Serious Side Effects:* Overdose, addiction, abuse.

## Medications to Treat/Prevent Extrapyramidal Symptoms (EPS)

Table 4-10. Medications for EPS

*Anticholinergics*

| Generic Name | Trade Name | Average Daily Dose | Notes/Precautions |
|---|---|---|---|
| benztropine | Cogentin | 1–6 mg | |
| biperiden | Akineton | 2–6 mg | |
| trihexyphenidyl | Artane | 1–10 mg | Should not be crushed |

*Antihistamines*

| Generic Name | Trade Name | Average Daily Dose | Notes/Precautions |
|---|---|---|---|
| diphenhydramine | Benadryl | 25–100 mg | |

*Dopamine Agonists*

| Generic Name | Trade Name | Average Daily Dose | Notes/Precautions |
|---|---|---|---|
| amantadine | Symmetrel | 100–300 mg | > parkinson |
| levodopa | Dopar | 500 mg–3000 mg | |

*Common Side Effects:* Dry mouth, sedation, blurred vision, constipation.

*Serious Side Effects:* Psychosis, toxicity.

## Central Nervous System (CNS) Stimulants

Use of CNS stimulants include: ADHD, narcolepsy, weight management, and refractory depression.

| Generic Name | Trade Name | Average Daily Dose | Notes/Precautions |
|---|---|---|---|
| amphetamine | Adderall | 5–30 mg | |
| d-amphetamine | Dexedrine | 5–30 mg | |
| methylphenidate | Ritalin | 5–40 mg | |
| pemoline | Cylert | 56.25–75 mg | |

*Common Side Effects:* Insomnia, anorexia, jitteriness, headaches.

*Serious Side Effects:* Tics, abuse, addiction, overdose, psychosis.

## Managing Side Effects of Psychotropic Medications

Side effects seen as a result of a patient taking psychotropic medications are generally produced by blockade receptors of muscarinic (cholinergic), alpha adrenergic, and histaminic receptors. (See Table 4-10)

### Muscarinic (Cholinergic)
Drying. Such adverse effects include: drying of mouth/lips.

### Histaminic H1 Receptor
Histamine functions by increasing gastric secretion, dilating capillaries, and constricting bronchial smooth muscles. Adverse effects seen as a result of blocking histamine are weight gain and sedation.

### Alpha-Adrenergic Receptor
It is a site in autonomic nerve pathways where the adrenergic receptors of epinephrine and norepinephrine are released and excitatory responses occur. An alpha-adrenergic blocking agent interferes with this transmission and will not allow sympathetic nervous excitatory stimuli to be effective. Adverse effects seen when the alpha-adrenergic receptor is blocked are: orthostatic hypotension, potentiation of antihypertensives, and reflex tachycardia.

### Dopamine D2 Receptor
Acts to increase blood pressure, especially systolic pressure, and increases urinary output. Side effects seen when the dopamine receptor is blocked are: prolactic elevation and extrapyramidal side effects.

### Table 4-11. Receptors and Side Effects

| Side Effect | Receptor Blockade | Intervention |
| --- | --- | --- |
| Blurred vision | Muscarinic (cholinergic) | Give patient reassurance. Most will subside in 2–6 weeks Ophthalmologist to be warned |
| Dry mouth and lips | Muscarinic (cholinergic) | Frequent sips of fluid Sugarless gum or hard candies Medication: bethanecol (Urecholine) |
| Constipation | Muscarinic (cholinergic) | High fiber diet Exercise Increase fluid intake Warm prune juice Mild laxative |
| Nasal congestion | Muscarinic (cholinergic) | Nose drops Moisturizer NOT nasal spray Assess for infections |
| Tachycardia | Muscarinic (cholinergic) | Reassurance May need to change medication |
| Speech and memory | Muscarinic (cholinergic) | May need to change medication Dysfunction |
| Urinary retention | Muscarinic (cholinergic) | Medication: Bethanecol |
| Vaginal dryness | Muscarinic (cholinergic) | Lubricants May need cholinergic medication |

(Continued on next page)

| Side Effect | Receptor Blockade | Intervention |
|---|---|---|
| Decreased libido/ anorgasmia | Adrenergic | Reassurance that it is reversible<br>Drug holiday<br>Use buproprion (Wellbutrin) |
| Edema | Adrenergic | Reassurance<br>Increase fluids and rest<br>May need diuretic |
| Postural hypotension | Adrenergic/histaminic | Obtain baseline vital signs<br>Instruct on slow position changes<br>Monitor BP with dosage changes<br>Instruct patient to pump feet prior<br>to sitting<br>May need to decrease dosage<br>Increase fluid intake |
| Drowsiness/sedation | Histaminic | Advise client to avoid dangerous<br>activities<br>Single dose at hs<br>Start gradually with sedating meds<br>Plan days to allow for rest if needed<br>Inform other health care givers<br>of psychotropic use<br>Be aware of interactions with<br>other sedating meds<br>If needed, switch to less sedating drug |
| Weight gain | Histaminic | Instruct regarding exercise and<br>low fat diet<br>Assess for fluid retention |
| Dermatitis | | Stop medication<br>Initiate comfort measures<br>Administer antihistamine |
| Exacerbation or attackof narrow-angle glaucoma | Muscarinic (cholinergic) | May need to adjust eye med or<br>change psychotropic drug |
| Photosensitivity | | Protective clothing: hats and long sleeves<br>Minimize sun exposure<br>Apply sun block SP15 or higher<br>Dark glasses<br>Lip sunblock<br>No tanning bed use<br>Apply wet/cool compresses<br>Change med to a nonphotosensitizing<br>alternative or decrease dosage |

(Continued on next page)

| Side Effect | Receptor Blockade | Intervention |
|---|---|---|
| Rhinitis (increased secretion of mucous) | | Encourage rest, adequate fluids |
| Impaired psychomotor functions | | Advise client to avoid dangerous activities. |
| Amenorrhea/ galactorrhea | Dopaminergic | Reassurance and counseling Lack of menses does not mean lack of ovulation Advise client to continue birth |
| control | | |
| Nausea/vomiting | | Reduce anxiety by methods of distraction Apply cool cloth to forehead, back of neck Suck on ice chips, eat clear soups, crackers, jello, dry toast, cooked cereal Avoid foods that are too hot or too cold Acupressure P6 point |

Side effect management from Merrie Kaas, DNSc, RN, CS; Sandy Seidel, MS, RN, CS; Beth Good, MS, RN, CS, CARN (1997).

## Neuroleptic Malignant Syndrome

Neuroleptic malignant syndrome (NMS) is a rare, but life-threatening adverse reaction to neuroleptic medications. Any D2 receptor antagonist medication can theoretically cause this reaction. The most common medications causing this reaction are typical antipsychotics. Typical high potency antipsychotics such as Haldol and Prolixin have a higher incidence. These medications are prescribed not only for psychosis and schizophrenia but for bipolar disorder, developmental disabilities, dementia, and nausea. The incidence of NMS is 0.5%, but the mortality rate is 10–20%. Death can occur in a matter of hours. Prompt detection and immediate medical intervention is indicated. Ninety percent of cases of NMS develop within 10 days after initiation of neuroleptic medications, but it can occur at any time during neuroleptic use.

Hallmark signs and symptoms of NMS are hyperthermia, diaphoresis, muscle rigidity, and confusion.

The patient is exhibiting autonomic dysregulation. The symptoms can vary from case to case. The diagnosis is made based on a cluster of symptoms. Unstable vital signs are exhibited. Not all patients exhibit all the classic symptoms. The diagnosis is often missed in the early stages. Symptoms evolve over 24 to 72 hours. Withdrawal or agitation may be mistakenly considered increased psychosis. Symptoms that can be present include:

- Hypertension
- Labile blood pressure
- Tachycardia

- A temperature above 100.4°F (38°C) degrees
- Muscle rigidity, quite severe or may be mild
- Tremor
- Incontinence
- Altered mental state ranging from confusion to coma; exhibiting disorientation
- Incontinence
- Dysphagia
- Pallor
- Mutism
- Abnormal labs
  - Elevated CPK
  - Leukocytosis
  - Elevated liver enzymes
  - Increased myoglobin in the plasma results in renal shutdown

The autonomic dysregulation is caused by dopamine receptor blockade causing rapid dopamine depletion of the hypothalamus. There is subsequent hyperthermia, diaphoresis, dehydration, and muscle rigidity. The muscle tissue breaks down causing rhabdomyolysis, exhibited by elevated CPK and myoglobin in the urine. Ultimately, without treatment, renal failure and death occur. In addition, the patient has respiratory and swallowing difficulties and may go into respiratory and/or cardiac arrest.

Several RISK FACTORS that place certain patients more at risk include:

- Prior adverse reactions to antipsychotic medications, including extrapyramidal reactions, dystonias, and Parkinsonian symptoms
- Dehydration and physical exhaustion
- An IM route of administration
- High dosages
- Rapid increase in dosage
- Being on two antipsychotics at once
- Patients with any concomitant organic brain syndrome

## Treatment of NMS

NMS is a medical emergency requiring immediate intervention. Immediately discontinue neuroleptic medications. Monitor all vital signs and treat the hyperthermia. Transfer the patient to an appropriate medical unit, probably the ICU. The patient needs IV hydration to correct volume depletion and correct fluid and electrolyte imbalance. The urine is alkalized with sodium bicarbonate ($NaHCO_3$). Dopamine agonist medications such as bromocriptine, apomorphine, amantadine, carbidopa, or levodopa are administered, usually IV. Dantrolene, a skeletal muscle relaxant, is given to decrease the breakdown of muscle tissue. Drug therapy favors bromocriptine over dantrolene. It is the most effective and safest treatment for NMS. Benzodiazepines are given to sedate the patient and heparin may be given to avoid embolism. Recovery may take 7–10 days or up to several weeks. Usually temperature, blood pressure instability, and CPK levels normalize in a few days. Recovery takes longer if the patient has had decanoate neuroleptics. The patient's psychiatric condition must be closely monitored during physical recovery.

Nursing errors have been the cause of death from unrecognized or inappropriately treated NMS. Always take the patient's medication history to see if there have been prior adverse reactions. This may require talking with family members. Record and notify the treating physician about any adverse reactions. Prominently display prior adverse reactions on the patient's chart. Monitor vital signs regularly of any hospitalized patients on neuroleptics. Ear thermometers are quite convenient for agitated or noncompliant patients. See that the patient has a physical exam, with labs, within 24 hours of admission to the hospital. Use astute clinical observation to ascertain confusion from psychotic symptoms. Withdraw neuroleptics and call the physician if the patient exhibits unstable BP, temperature above 100.4°F (38°C), rigidity, or significant confusion. Always be sure there is a crash cart on the unit (Rother, 2001).

## Serotonin Syndrome

Serotonin syndrome includes the following symptoms:
- Altered mental status
- Diaphoresis
- Diarrhea
- Fever
- Hyperreflexia
- Incoordination
- Muscular rigidity
- Shivering
- Tremors

Serotonin syndrome can develop within several hours, but can also take weeks. It generally resolves within 24 hours. It is thought to be due to the hyperstimulation of the serotonin system. Any type of drug that increases serotonin transmission can be a possible offender.

### Treatment
Stop medications immediately. Use supportive measures such as IV fluids, cooling blanket, antipyretics.

## Prescriptive Authority for the Clinical Specialist in Psychiatric and Mental Health Nursing

In order for the APPN to prescribe medication, the CNS must:

- have a master's degree;
- be certified as a clinical specialist in psychiatric and mental health nursing by the American Nurses Credentialing Center;
- have successfully completed at least 30 hours of formal study in pharmacology consistent with the course requirements outlined in the law; and
- have a collaborative agreement with a psychiatrist or physician, based on standards established by your state nurses association and the state psychiatric society.

Prescriptive practice authority granted to nurses is generally the result of a statute (an act of the legislature) or through regulations and rules declared by state agencies (generally medical or nursing boards) that have the power and authority to adopt such rules (Hadley, 1990). These laws vary from state to state. Some states require nurse practitioner licensure before nurses can prescribe.

There are two common types of prescriptive authority:

1. **Complementary authority** is the arrangement where the nurse must have a collaborating physician (in most cases a psychiatrist) and a plan for supervision. Complementary authority is less autonomous than substitutive authority (Hadley, 1989).

2. **Substitutive authority** is where the nurse is able to prescribe medication without the supervision of a physician (or psychiatrist) (Talley & Brooke, 1992).

## Electroconvulsive Therapy (ECT)

ECT remains one of the most powerful and controversial treatments in psychiatry. With refinements in technique and usages, ECT today is a strong presence in the armament to fight mental illnesses. It is most commonly used to treat refractory major depression.

## Historical Perspective

ECT was first introduced in 1937 in Rome based on the later disproved theory that there was a "biological antagonism" between severe psychiatric disorders and epilepsy. It was initially used for schizophrenia and other serious mental illnesses. Psychotropic medications were not available until well into the 1950s. Until then ECT, psychosurgery (such as lobotomies and trephination), physical restraint and/or seclusion, hydrotherapy, and insulin coma were the only alternatives. Given these facts, ECT was used quite extensively. At that time, neuromuscular blockade was not available and general anesthetics were not administered when ECT was performed. The patient was manually restrained and there were at times broken bones and bitten tongues. These factors led to ECT's poor reputation and its restricted use today.

## ECT Today

ECT today is a good choice for some patients. We know so very much more now about the diagnoses and biology of mental illnesses. We have learned the safest and most efficacious ways to administer ECT. We have learned the proper indications for ECT. Meanwhile, the area of psychopharmacology has grown exponentially. Today ECT is used only as a secondary or tertiary alternative treatment after multiple trials of medications (Calev, 1994; Glass, 2001).

## Indications

Indications for the use of ECT are: refractory major depression, severe catatonic withdrawal, and acute possiblity of suicidal behavior. It is most commonly used and is most effective for refractory major depression. Additionally, some patients with bipolar affective disorder or acute schizophrenia who are unresponsive to appropriate trials of psychotropic medications may benefit from a course of ECT. It has also been used in acute mania when the patient is at risk of exhaustion and not responding to other measures. Some patients who have OBS with psychosis from arteriosclerosis or senility may show symptomatic behavior improvement following ECT. A previous good response to ECT or a family history of positive ECT response may predict a good response to ECT. If a patient is acutely suicidal or catatonic, ECT might be preferred because the patient may respond faster than to medications. ECT can have some other advantages over psychopharmacology for certain patients. If the patient is nonresponsive or hypersensitive to medications or if she is pregnant, ECT may be the safer choice. It can be safer and better tolerated than medications for many older adult patients and is often used in the older adult. There is a 50–60% response rate to ECT for patients who have not responded to one or more trials of antidepressant therapy. ECT has *not* been found to be effective for neuroses, thought disorders, individuality disorders, or grief reactions.

## Precautions and Contraindications

Patients with acute heart disease or aortic aneurisms would not be good candidates. Someone with pneumonia may not tolerate the required anesthesia. The mortality rate of ECT is 1 in 10,000 treatments. This is lower than for patients having surgery with general anesthesia and in spite of the high percentage of older adults receiving this treatment. Patients have been successfully treated with ECT who have known cardiovascular disease, peptic ulcers, and glaucoma. A brain tumor is an absolute contraindication, because the increases in intracranial pressure during a convulsion may lead to brainstem herniation and cause the death of a client with a preexisting elevated pressure.

## Mechanism of Action

ECT is an electrically induced grand mal seizure. The therapeutic effect is thought to be the result of an alteration in the postsynaptic response to the neurotransmitters in the central nervous system. ECT stimulates synaptic remodeling—the number of vesicles that contain synaptic protein increases, producing an enhanced behavioral response and relief from depressive symptoms.

## The Procedure

First and foremost, consent is crucial. In California, two psychiatrists must concur and the patient must have had two adequate trials of two categories of antidepressants. A signed consent from the patient must be obtained and can be rescinded verbally at any time. In rare cases where a patient is conserved, the conservator and a judge may order ECT if all the other criteria for treatment are met. These rules vary from state to state.

The procedure is usually performed in the OR suite of the hospital and anesthesia is administered by an anesthesiologist. The nursing care is similar to a surgical procedure. ECT has previously been performed in a treatment room on the psychiatric ward with the psychiatrist administering the anesthesia and a specially trained nurse in attendance. This is still the case in some institutions. Emergency equipment is always readily available wherever the procedure is performed. The patient is NPO after midnight. Jewelry and dentures are removed and the patient should empty his/her bladder. Displaying a confident attitude toward the patient's choice and the procedure will reduce the patient's apprehension.

During the procedure, the patient must be ventilated and their vital signs and IV monitored. Oxygen is administered to decrease postictal confusion and memory loss. The medications used are methohexital (Brevital) 5–10 ml of 10 mg/ml IV solution, a short acting barbiturate used to induce sleep, and succinylcholine chloride (Anectine) 0.3–5 ml of 20 mg/ml solution, a short acting skeletal muscle relaxant causing flaccid paralysis. The onset is rapid and the effect lasts 4-6 minutes. These induce unconsciousness and neuromuscular blockade.

An electrical stimulus of 70–150 volts to the brain for 0.1–1 second is then administered to produce a grand mal seizure. The seizure lasts 30–60 seconds only and is evidenced by EEG or by observation of rhythmic movements of the distal digits. Movements are slight and often limited to plantar flexion of the feet followed by rhythmic twitching of the toes.

There is controversy in the literature and in practice regarding bilateral vs. unilateral electrode placement. Unilateral ECT, application of the electrical current to the patient's nondominant hemisphere, is thought to cause less cognitive adverse effects. Some clinicians believe that bilateral ECT is more efficacious. One approach is to begin the series with unilateral electrode placement and switch to bilateral after about six treatments if there has been no response.

A full course of ECT treatment typically consists of 3 treatments per week for 2–6 weeks, depending on the response of the patient. It is usually done on an inpatient but can be done on an outpatient basis. As the patient gets better, he or she may be able to go home but return to the hospital 2–3 times per week for the rest of the course of treatment. Patients often have an initial response after the first few treatments, but the full course is still necessary to achieve complete remission from the depression.

## Post-Procedure Care

The patient's vital signs must be monitored frequently. Each hospital has a set protocol. Postural hypotension is common and drowsiness is normal. Check for orientation and alertness. Observe for signs of confusion. Reorient and reassure the patient. Make sure the patient is hydrated and fed a light breakfast. Typically, the patient is fully responsive in about 15 minutes and fully recovered in 1–2 hours. Documentation of the patient's mental and physical responses, during and after the treatment, is an important nursing duty.

## Adverse Effects

The main risks of ECT are those posed by undergoing general anesthesia. The main adverse reactions to ECT itself are cognitive. Postictal confusion and short-term memory loss are the most common. The immediate confusion clears in a few minutes to hours. Most often there is short-term memory loss that worsens towards the end of the series and then improves in the weeks after cessation of treatments. Neuropsychological studies consistently have shown that by several months after the completion of ECT, the ability to learn and remember is normal. Rarely, patients can have permanent loss of memory for events that occurred in the period just preceding the course of therapy (retrograde amnesia).

## Conjoint and Follow-Up Care

Since depression is a recurrent condition in 50% of the cases and has a high mortality rate, most patients need ongoing treatment. If a patient can tolerate and is responsive to antidepressants, they are the choice for therapy following ECT. However, these are the more difficult to treat patients who have often had multiple medication trials and failures prior to ECT. A patient may have been so acutely ill that he or she needed the immediacy of ECT, but afterwards a new medication regimen may work. Some patients are given maintenance ECT, a treatment about once a month to avoid a relapse into severe depression. Supportive psychotherapy—both group and individual, along with psychoeducation—is important in the overall treatment of the patient. The family should be involved in the treatment if at all possible.

## Summary

Electroconvulsive therapy has a place in the therapies we use to treat mental illnesses, especially life-threatening and debilitating depression. A psychiatric nurse must be knowledgeable about the correct indications for ECT, including the potential benefits and risks. The nurse must be competent in the nursing care required before, during, and after the procedure. The nurse must also know the appropriate conjoint and follow-up care and treatment required to treat the mental illness for which the patient is receiving ECT.

## Biofeedback

Biofeedback is the therapeutic technique of using equipment, usually electronic, to reveal internal physiological events. Feedback is in the form of visual and auditory signals. The goal is to teach an individual to manipulate involuntary events through the feedback signals. The assumption is that the autonomic nervous system can be instrumentally conditioned.

For biofeedback to work it must be possible to detect and accurately measure the desired physiological activity. There also must be a flow of continuous or near-continuous information fed back to the patient and the patient must be motivated to learn. Types of feedback used are the galvanic skin response, heart rate, blood pressure, temperature, electromyogram (EMG), and electroencephalogram (EEG).

There are several ways to measure whether the desired learning took place. Is the patient able to control the parameter measured in the presence of the biofeedback signal? Is the patient able to demonstrate control of the parameter without the signal? Are there changes in the initial resting baseline across sessions? Is the patient able to demonstrate the ability to control the parameter in a variety of settings? And is there maintenance of the response across time?

## Phototherapy

The use of phototherapy in seasonal depression has been well established. Phototherapy consists of the application of light to the eyes at a predetermined intensity and duration. Light intensity is measured in *lux*. Phototherapy in seasonal depression usually consists of morning exposure of 2500 lux for a period of approximately an hour. Melatonin is produced in darkness, and as the days of late autumn and winter progress, melatonin production increases to abnormally high levels in some individuals. The notion that light suppresses melatonin is a critical notion. Suppressing melatonin production reverses the symptoms. It is effective in approximately 60% of individuals with seasonally related symptoms.

Phototherapy has also been reported by some to have efficacy in nonseasonal depression. The use of phototherapy to augment the effects of medication for individuals who are partial responders has shown some promise. There has also been some study of the use of phototherapy to adjust disturbed sleep/wake cycles.
(Beck, Rawlins, & Williams, 1993)

## Group Therapy

Group therapy is a powerful healing technique with several different formats. The basic premises of group therapy are: 1) that human beings are social animals, and 2) that we heal in community. This is why group therapy is so efficacious. This correlates to Maslow's third level in his hierarchy of needs; the need for love and belonging. The importance of social support has been studied extensively. Group therapy provides a valuable form of social support, especially for isolated individuals such as the chronically mentally ill or combat veterans. Ideally, the individual also has other forms of social support. Group is a microcosm of society and the family. In group therapy, we create a small society. One's family of origin is one's primary group and this is recreated in group therapy.

Group therapy is not something to be undertaken lightly. Group therapists should be trained in and have knowledge of many theories and techniques. The dynamics of human social behavior, psychopathology, group process, and experience with a variety of group therapy techniques are essential before leading group therapy sessions. Therapists and co-therapists should have experience in a group as a participant as part of their training.

Group therapy training conferences are available throughout the country. Usually these are experiential where the participant is the future therapist. Observing group therapy is another valuable learning tool. Most teaching institutions have this available to nursing students, often with a post evaluation session with the group therapist. This is an excellent way to begin learning. Clinical supervision is also useful and necessary. There are several characteristics, including a "healthy narcissism," that make a good group therapist:

- Reflects a stable sense of one's worth based on realistic achievement.
- Has the ability to recover quickly from disappointment and failure.
- Finds reassurance and support in one's relationships when needed.
- Pays attention to the client's needs and also to self-interest.
- Does not feel he or she must be available to clients no matter what the cost.
- Knows that psychiatric work is not characterized by easy successes or immediate gratification.
- Able to tolerate ambiguity.
- Knows that whatever unfolds in treatment is completely expected.

A co-leader is necessary for most groups, unless the group is very small and the patients are well known to the therapist. The co-leader serves many purposes, such as sharing different perspectives, picking up emotions from patients that may be missed by one therapist, and providing a needed balance of energies. The leader and co-leader can also cover for each other should one or the other need to be absent, thereby allowing the group to meet. The leader and the co-leader must spend time together discussing their techniques, their patients, and most importantly the relationship between the two of them. The leaders must be in unison or the group can become very dysfunctional.

As each individual is unique, each group is unique. On any given day, a group is unique from the last session, even with the same members present. Each group should have established ground rules developed by the participants with guidance from the leaders. These ground rules need to be developed early on and they will vary from group to group. They can be adapted as new members join and as different issues surface. These rules establish boundaries and may take a few sessions to develop. Time will be needed to reevaluate these ground rules on a regular basis.

Irving Yalom (1983, 1985) is a renowned group therapist. He employs two types of groups—the agenda group and the focus group; these will be discussed. He has identified eleven curative factors of group therapy.

- *Imparting information:* This is receiving didactic information and advice. We educate the patients and the patients educate each other. Topics such as psychopharmacology, medical issues, financial and insurance resources are often discussed.

- *Instillation of HOPE:* When a individual sees another who is getting better or coping it gives them hope, and this is healing and curative.

- *Universality:* Gives the knowledge that they are not alone and the realization that others have the same feelings, thoughts, and problems as they have. Be it breast cancer, chemical dependency, hallucinations, homicidal or suicidal thoughts, or depression, the concept is the same: "We are not alone."

- *Altruism:* Underrated important facet of human behavior. We feel good when we do good for others. We want to do good for others. In group, when you help another it helps you to heal your own issues and pain. It is the ability to forget ourselves and become absorbed in someone or something outside of ourselves.

- *Corrective reenactment of the primary family group:* The ability of members to alter learning experiences previously obtained in their family of origin. It is an opportunity to try interacting in a different way.

- *Development of social interaction techniques:* The opportunity to develop new skills and to increase one's awareness of social interactions.

- *Imitative behaviors:* Opportunity to increase skills by imitating behaviors of others in the group, such as not interrupting or monopolizing.

- *Interindividual learning:* Ability to engage in wider range of interindividual exchanges, thereby increasing each member's understanding of responsibility and complexity of interindividual relationships and decreasing members' interindividual distortions. Opportunity to check reality with a number of individuals. The individual also learns how he or she is perceived by other individuals.

- *Existential Factors:* Why am I here? What is the meaning of my existence? Why do bad things happen? Why do individuals die? Group provides an opportunity in a safe environment to discuss these issues and gain perspective.

- *Catharsis:* Opportunity to express feelings in a safe, appropriate environment. Okay to be angry, but not physically violent. Okay to cry, but not to inflict harm on self. A release of suppressed emotions.

- *Group cohesion:* This is vital for the group to stay together. There has to be a common bond, an attraction to each other, and a commitment to the group. This provides a sense of belonging as well.

Yalom's group agenda is for higher functioning patients. The agenda group size is from 6–12 patients, either inpatient or outpatient. The group runs 1–1.5 hours. Each individual states an agenda for that day's session and is asked if he or she wants time to work during the session or not. Then members work one at a time. Not all members will work each session. At the end of the group, all members share what the work done that day has brought up for them and how it ties in with their particular agenda for that day. This is not advice, but rather a reflection on how the issues discussed relate to their own life issues.

The focus group that Yalom describes is for lower functioning patients and is smaller. Four to seven patients is ideal. There is more pathology in the room and the patients require more individual attention and direction. These patients may be actively psychotic or severely depressed or anxious. They are usually hospitalized. The goal is to make this a successful, non-anxiety-producing experience so that the patient begins to feel comfortable coming to group therapy. This type of group provides human contact in a safe, structured, secure environment. The group length is shorter, typically 45 minutes, to accommodate the shorter attention span of these patients. There should be a consistent leader. The leader must also be very flexible. The assistance of a co-leader is very helpful. Simple tasks that the patients can succeed in doing are used regularly. Such things as drawing a picture or sharing a recent nonthreatening event, like a meal, might be done. Positive reinforcement should be used generously.

There are many types and forms of groups. Marram describes a continuum of group therapy that is a useful model. Groups range from support groups to individuality reconstruction groups. Support groups reinforce the group members' healthier defenses. The self-help groups like Alcoholics Anonymous, which are so effective in treating chemical dependency, are an example of this. Remotivation and reeducation groups increase communication and interaction among members. These groups help members to learn more socially appropriate and adaptive behaviors. Social activities such as outings might be employed.

Problem-solving groups focus on a specific problem and on problem-solving techniques. The group is usually time limited. An example might be a task force at the hospital to solve a quality assurance issue. Insight and reconstruction groups emphasize interindividual communication and focus on goals of alleviating emotional stress and affecting change by increasing the individual's cognitive and emotional understanding of his problems. This is the most typical form of group therapy.

Individuality reconstruction groups go to an even deeper level using psychoanalytical theory and unconscious material. Such techniques as dream analysis may be used. The goal is for group members to increase understanding of their individualities and defensive structures and to modify their behavioral and defensive patterns.

*Psychodrama*, as defined by Jacob Moreno, is a group therapy technique in which individuals express their emotional problems through play acting or drama. It should only be done by a trained therapist and with higher functioning patients. Emotions surface quickly and the therapist and co-therapist must be ready to respond. The patient working is designated as the protagonist. The therapist is the director. Auxiliary egos are other group members portraying characters in the protagonist's drama. The audience consists of the other group members.

There are several techniques employed during this process. Soliloquy is when the protagonist talks to themselves while being observed by the group. Role reversal is allowing the protagonist to play other, conflicting roles, and also using alter egos to play protagonist. Mirroring takes place when the alter egos imitate the protagonist in an attempt to allow him to see how others see him. Closure is an important process at the end of the group. Every group member shares his or her observations and shares back what the drama brought up for each of them. Closure for the protagonist is especially important.

Any time individuals join together, it is a group. Informal social interactions are a group. Education groups are very important. These can be experiential or didactic. Family members can be invited to educational groups. Psychopharmacology educational groups are valuable.

Stress management and assertiveness training are useful group techniques. Twelve-step groups are unique and powerful. The success rate for recovery from addiction is quite high with activity in 12-step programs. They are also readily available and free of charge.

Attend meetings in your community to become familiar with the format. A speaker shares and specifies a topic, then individuals share sequentially. There is no feedback or discussion during the meeting. Individual issues are discussed one on one. This is discussed more thoroughly in this manual in the chemical dependency section.

## Family Therapy

Every patient comes from a family. Most family therapists employ the concepts of general systems theory to work with the family as a system. Communication techniques and styles within the family are also a foundation of working with families. Ackerman, Whittaker, Minuchin, and Bowen are the main family systems theorists and therapists. Satir and Haley focus on communication techniques and styles in families.

When the family is viewed as a system, there are some basic definitions agreed upon by family therapists. The family is the **system**. The **subsystems** are defined as **parental, spousal**, and **sibling**. Varying types of **boundaries** exist between these subsystems and between the family and society. Boundaries are defined as **loose, rigid**, or **permeable**. The individual in the family who is the "sick" one or the one with the problem is the **identified patient** (IP). In fact, this individual may not be the one with the most pathology in the family and his or her behavior can often be viewed as adaptive, functional, and purposive within the individual's environment, e.g., the family system.

As in all systems, **homeostasis** is a strong drive, so change takes effort and time. Families have ranges of acceptable and familiar change or movement. The family will create and use a scapegoat to regain balance or homeostasis. A triangle evolves out of twosomes that are inherently unstable. The third individual of the triangle absorbs the anxiety. This is termed **triangulation**, and the individual triangulated is usually the IP.

**Family myths** are incorrect beliefs about family history. They usually exist in covert form and function to maintain the status quo. Every family has overt and covert **family rules** as well. The **nuclear family** is the immediate family in the household. The **extended family** is the entire family. Families develop through a series of phases: courtship, early marriage, expansion, consolidation, contraction, final partnership, and disappearance of family.

An agreed-upon goal of family systems therapy is **differentiation** of the self from the family ego mass so that each individual can achieve full potential. Each member of a couple must differentiate from their family of origin before the couple starts their own family. Compulsive marital repetition occurs when the parents' marriage is repeated with accuracy. The individuals of the couple must be at the same level of differentiation for homeostasis to be present. Some symptoms of undifferentiation in marriage are: marital conflict, dysfunction in one spouse, and projection of problems onto a child.

A family that is **enmeshed** is one with very loose boundaries around the individuals. Individuals have very little autonomy or individuality. A family that is **disengaged** has very rigid boundaries between the individuals. The boundary between the family and society must be evaluated. Family dysfunction has many forms. Often an enmeshed family has a rigid boundary between itself and society. This cuts off the family from society and can be the setting for such problems as incest and eating disorders. A disengaged family often has loose boundaries between itself and society and the "family" is more like a group of roommates. There is little or no oneness among the family members. There is often little supervision of children and acting-out behavior in adolescents can occur in this type of family.

Families that have permeable boundaries are the most functional, because they provide flexibility and an environment where each individual is treated uniquely and there is a healthy interchange between the family and society. Family members feel a sense of oneness with the family and are also able to experience individuality. Family therapy intervention is designed to alleviate multiple interlocking emotional disorders of the family group. Goals of therapy include facilitating communications of thoughts and feelings in order to shift disturbed, inflexible roles and coalitions within the family.

The first order of business for the family therapist(s) is to establish rapport, empathy, and communication. Often family therapy is done with two co-therapists, male and female. The therapists serve as role models, educators, and de-mythologizers. The therapist's role is to offer reeducation, reorganization through communication change, and a resolution of pathogenic conflict. The therapist uses this rapport to catalyze expression of major conflicts. Introducing a significant other individual (the therapist) into a disturbed family system has the capacity to modify relationships within the system.

The therapist counteracts inappropriate denial, displacements, and rationalizations. He/she transforms dormant concealed interindividual conflicts into open, interactional expression. This neutralizes the process of prejudicial scapegoating and fulfills, in part, the role of a real parent figure. The therapist also continues with the roles of educator and role model. To keep the family returning for therapy, it is helpful for the therapist to side with the individual in power while attributing positive qualities to the individual most likely to return to therapy.

To further the goal of differentiation of self, the therapist works towards shifting the emotional cutoff in the family system. The greater the intensity of the emotional cutoff from the family of origin, the more vulnerable the individual is to duplicate marital and family patterns. This can be an unconscious way of working through the unresolved issues. It can be beneficial to reestablish emotional contact with the family of origin. This can reduce anxiety and symptoms, but the individual may need therapeutic help to avoid making things worse and for support and guidance while going through the process. When emotional contact is maintained in a healthy fashion, it promotes health in the current and future generations. The goal can be to move from an intense emotional cutoff from the family of origin to at least an average relationship of formality with some distance and returning home for duty visits.

Some family therapy techniques are supervisory. The therapist essentially "coaches" the family members on working within their own family. The therapist functions by defining and clarifying the relationship between spouses, keeps himself from being triangulated in the family emotional system, teaches the function of the emotional system, and demonstrates differentiation by taking an "I" position at varying times throughout the therapy.

Minuchin has a specific technique called structural therapy. He works with families by shifting their structure and allowing them to operate in new ways. The transactional patterns are analyzed and then the system is stressed by changing the structure, sometimes literally the geographical structure, in a session. Then individual boundaries are clearly delineated for and with the family. The therapist actively blocks usual communication patterns and helps the family to develop different channels of communication. Homework is often assigned. The purpose of the IP's symptoms in the family is focused on and clarified. The therapist re-labels the symptoms for the family. Eventually the enmeshments are untangled and the boundaries clear.

Satir and Haley both work with families around communication techniques. Satir describes the way individuals under stress handle their communication. The **placater** agrees, apologizes, and wants to please. The **blamer** finds fault and is dominant and accusatory. The **computer** is the one who communicates when stressed by being reasonable, calm, and emotionally detached. Some individuals relate by bringing up irrelevant subjects as a way to distract from the stress. **Congruent** communication is the healthiest. This is when a individual communicates in a genuine manner using straight, expressive messages. Haley adds that when communication is ineffective the symptoms of the IP become the covert message. Often the family members, especially the children, can be placed in a classic double bind where they can neither confront nor leave the dysfunctional situation. The goal is to teach the family to communicate clearly and identify feelings so that the dysfunctional behaviors or symptoms can change.

## Sex Therapy

Sex is an important part of family life. If a couple is experiencing sexual dysfunction, marital satisfaction diminishes and the family unit suffers. Sex therapy can be beneficial in this situation. Masters and Johnson and Helen Kaplan are leaders in the arena of sex therapy. Sexual dysfunctions can be related to one or more causes. Physical reasons must be ruled out first. If medical issues are found, then current pharmacological and surgical interventions can be very successful. Performance anxiety, religious/moral inhibitions, or fear of losing control can contribute to sexual difficulties. Sometimes there is a lack of educative information and/or communication. Unrealistic expectations can also interfere with sexual functioning.

The rational application of structured sexual experiences to treat sexual dysfunction is the strategy employed by Masters and Johnson as well as Kaplan. The goal is for each individual to act on his or her own behalf and for both partners to achieve mutual sexual satisfaction. Homework exercises are prescribed for the couple by the therapist. The aim of the homework exercises is to shift the couple's objective away from the achievement of a response to the giving and receiving of pleasure. Their attention is thus diverted and focused on the experience of erotic feelings in an effort to modify the destructive tendency to stand apart and to observe oneself and to judge the sexual experience on the basis of one's ability to produce a performance. The couple is helped to combat the tendency toward playing spectator of the sexual performance.

To prolong pleasuring and endurance, the couple is taught a start-stop exercise of stopping sexual activity just before the point of inevitability and then resuming activity. The couple takes turns and each partner is encouraged towards selfishness. The giving and receiving of pleasurable sensual stimulation that does not ultimately lead to coitus is practiced. The therapist acts as a catalyst and facilitator to the couple's growth and change. As soon as possible the therapist turns responsibility over to the couple.

## Individual Therapies

### Behavioral Therapy

Isaac Pavlov and B.F. Skinner are the founders of behavioral therapy. The basic premise is that all behavior is learned and can therefore be modified through systematic manipulations of environmental variables. The goals are to create new learning or new behaviors and/or to remove or replace undesirable behaviors.

There are some basic principles involved. First, a problem behavior or a desired behavior must be identified. A way to measure it must be identified, such as time, frequency, or duration. Goals and objectives must be clearly stated in these measurable terms. Then an intervention plan must be devised. During the intervention period, competing behaviors are no longer rewarded and the desired behavior is rewarded. Then the interventions are phased out and the behavior should still be present. Ongoing checks for relapses of the unwanted behavior or to see if the desired behavior is continued is done periodically.

Specific techniques are employed to increase or decrease behaviors. **Shaping** is to train by gradually adding more parts to the task, like learning a dance routine and adding a few more steps each time to the combination. The concept of **successive approximation** is involved here as well. The behavior does not have to be done perfectly in the beginning to receive the reward, but over time this approximation gets closer and eventually becomes the desired behavior. **Extinction** is decreasing a behavior by removing rewards that maintain the behavior, like not laughing when a child misbehaves.

**Modeling** is learning the desired behavior by observing a competent model and imitating him or her. **Punishment** is inhibiting an undesirable response by making punishment contingent upon it, like grounding a teenager. **Toleration method** or **systematic desensitization** is used to deal with fears. Gradually the individual is exposed to the feared object while counter-conditioning of relaxation is performed. **Stimulus control** is controlling cues that prompt the behavior, like helping a individual with PTSD to identify triggers and to avoid them.

### Patient-Centered Therapy

Carl Rogers developed a therapeutic approach that is nondirective and stems from secular humanism. His assumption is that individuals are basically good and the goal of therapy is self-actualization. He believes that an inherent tendency in all organisms is to grow towards fulfillment and that this growth potential is best released in a relationship that contains empathy, genuineness, and unconditional positive regard. It is the therapist as a human being that is the remedy, not the technical skill. A troubled individual is someone whose self-concept has become structured in ways that are incongruent with organismic experience. In other words, there are inconsistencies between the organismic self and the conscious self.

The therapeutic approach is nondirective. The patient decides what to talk about, when, and when to end, the concept being that individuals themselves are the best source for their own answers. Unconditional positive regard is, according to Rogers, the most healing force in the universe. The therapist must avoid any behavior that is overtly or covertly judgmental. Genuineness is the absolute foundation for any healing relationship.

Certain techniques are employed in Rogerian therapy. **Structuring** is specific in patient-centered therapy. The patient is responsible for what is discussed during therapy and the therapist does not ask or answer questions. The therapy is structured by general leads; these include a brief introduction and the switch of responsibility back to the patient. **Defining limits** is the therapist's refusal to be manipulated by the patient. **Handling silence** is also the patient's responsibility. If the patient chooses to spend time in silence, it is the patient's choice. **Pacing** is tracking the patient's speed, tone, nonverbal expression, and body language. This demonstrates that the therapist is in tune with the patient. **Acceptance** is demonstrated in several ways. **Verbal reflection** is capturing the message of the patient in a fresh new way. By reflecting affect as well as content, the therapist shows empathy. **Nonverbal mirroring** is picking up the main cues and messages and communicating concern, attention, and interest. **Active listening** shows the therapist is attentive by vocal assent, eye contact, head nodding, etc. The use of **reflection** in varying forms is predominant.

## Cognitive Therapy

Developed by Aaron Beck, cognitive therapy is based on the philosophy that individuals can learn to be their own therapist. Emphasis is on the rearrangement of a individual's maladaptive processes of thinking, perception, and attitudes utilizing an active, time-limited approach. The basic assumption is that distorted thinking contributes to and maintains behavior (symptoms). The goal of the therapy is to limit the severity and debilitating aspects of symptoms (Beck, 1979).

There are certain basic principles of cognitive therapy. The foundation is that thinking is learned and can be changed. Further, negative thinking makes problem solving difficult and different thinking can lead to changed emotions. There is a link between THOUGHTS-EMOTIONS-BEHAVIORS. The patient learns to monitor his or her negative automatic thoughts to recognize the connection between cognition, affect, and behavior. Patients examine the evidence logically for and against their distorted automatic thinking and substitute more reality-oriented interpretations for their biased cognitions. They are then able to identify and alter dysfunctional beliefs that predispose them to distort their experiences.

Often the therapist gives written assignments to the patient; this therapy is usually time limited. Patients measure maladaptive emotions and beliefs initially and then at regular intervals. Patients are taught methods to discover how certain types of thinking make them feel. Specific self-verbalizations are used as guidelines as are reinforcing self-statements. Objective feedback is provided through measurement tools and journals logging thoughts, emotions, and behaviors. The therapist trains patients to recognize spontaneous verbal and pictorial cognitions (automatic thoughts). Patients report thoughts and images in detail. These spontaneous cognitions are then used to pinpoint patients' misconceptions to reality-test their distorted view of themselves and their world.

Steps in this therapy might include:

• Recognize your own automatic thoughts whenever you feel anxious.
• Keep track of these in a notebook.

- Develop and carry out strategies for testing your thoughts.
- Discuss your results.
- Role-play or practice.

## Gestalt Therapy

Frederick "Fritz" Perls developed Gestalt therapy. Gestalt treats "the whole individual." Perls assumes that we are born with an innate capacity to deal with life. And he believes that the past, such as habits, resentments, and unfinished business, is always present yet we must speak and act in concurrence with the here and now. Whether the future is thought of with hope or dread is important. The individual must be understood in the context of his or her ongoing relationship with the environment. *The goal of Gestalt therapy is greater awareness in all areas at any given moment, thus acquiring more internal regulation.*

The processes one must go through to achieve the desired goal are awareness, acceptance, and assimilation. Several powerful techniques are employed to facilitate this process. The most widely known is use of the empty chair. The patient puts anyone he wants in an empty chair opposite him and has a dialogue. The patient also moves into the empty chair and becomes the individual he is talking with. The empty chair can hold a "significant other" of the patient. It can also hold facets of the patient's individuality that are in conflict. Repeating, intensifying, and preserving emotions is done to help the patient experience intense emotions in a safe environment and learn to deal with them.

Fantasy and free association are also frequently used. The concepts of top dog and underdog are used to help an individual see the roles he plays in different situations and with different individuals. The patient is taught awareness of giving over power and allowing oneself to be used. The patient is also helped to become aware of rules he abides by unconsciously. The concept of positive withdrawal is introduced. Positive withdrawal is psychic withdrawal from an unhealthy relationship, enabling a patient to maintain power.

Gestalt therapy, when done correctly, is quite effective and powerful. The patient must be in a high functioning state to utilize this therapy effectively, and it should be done with compassion and as designed.

## Hypnosis

Hypnosis is a form of induced concentration with diminished peripheral awareness. A psychiatrist or therapist with specialized training and credentials generally conducts it. F.A. Mesmer devised the concept, thus the term "mesmerized." Spiegel and Spiegel, father and son who are both psychiatrists, are the most well-known hypnotists in the US. Hypnosis can be used for a variety of reasons. It can be used for regressive therapy to gain insights into past or recent traumatic events. It is most commonly used for behavior modification in the areas of smoking, eating disorders, weight control, anxiety, phobias, and pain control.

The technique is preformed in a quiet, relaxed, and safe environment. The therapist allows time for or already has established rapport with the patient. The hypnotizability of the patient is determined. This includes biological and psychological factors. Paranoid and suspicious individuals are typically not good candidates. If the patient is found to be a good candidate, mutual goals are then determined before the onset of hypnosis. Essentially all hypnosis is self-hypnosis, because it is the patient who puts himself in the trance. Therefore, it is essential that the goal of the hypnosis be identified by the patient. There are three levels of trance: light (motor retardation), medium (partial amnesia, anesthesia), and deep (post-hypnotic suggestion, age regression). To induce the trance state, the patient makes himself comfortable and concentrates. He then abandons executive control and submits to a dissociated state. The therapist is the coach towards this end. What occurs varies widely depending on the subject, the hypnotist, and their expectations.

# Crisis Intervention

Gerald Caplan, a pioneer in crisis intervention, described crisis as a state that occurs when one's usual ways of coping are inadequate to deal with the stress. Caplan emphasizes that crisis is characteristically self-limiting and lasts 4–6 weeks. Maximum goal is improvement of functioning above the pre-crisis level. There are three types of crises:

*Situational:* Specific external event upsets equilibrium.
*Maturational:* Occurs at transition points in aging (see Erikson).
*Adventitious:* Accidental, unexpected.

## Characteristics of the Crisis State
When individuals are unable to solve some significant problem in their lives, they:
- begin to experience tension and anxiety;
- have a decline in their overall functioning;
- develop somatic complaints;
- experience perceptual changes and intense feelings, e.g., sense of urgency, "going crazy," hallucinations; and
- have impaired impulse control.

They are frequently isolated from their usual sources of help (support system).

## Three Phases of Crisis Intervention
1. *Developing an alliance*
- Build trust, utilize empathy.
- Begin where the client wants to begin.
- Acknowledge feelings of helplessness.

2. *Gathering information*
- Focus on the precipitating event: "What is going on?" and "Why now, rather than two days ago?"
- Have there been similar symptoms in the past?
- Have there been similar stressors or situations in the past?
- How did you cope with them in the past?
- Why is the individual susceptible to this stress at this time?
- What and where are the usual resources?
- What was the previous level of functioning?

3. *Problem solving*
- Early formulation—begin some basic problem solving immediately.
- Set realistic goals.
- What does the client want?
- Focus on termination from the start.
- Support positive strengths.

• Avoid advice.
• Team approach.

## Identifying Difficult Behavior

Difficult behavior is what patients do despite corrective feedback from their nurse/healthcare giver. Difficult behavior is behavior that is hard to understand or solve. Difficult behavior is behavior that is troublesome and/or worrisome to the nurse.

"Difficult Patient Situations" evolve as a three-step process:

1.  A situation happens (e.g., a diabetic patient compulsively eats sugar; an alcoholic patient hides liquor in his hospital room; a chemically dependent patient is discharged from the mental health unit and is found stealing used syringes and using them).

2.  You react to the situation.
    •   Have thoughts about what just happened.
    •   Have feelings about what you think just happened.
    •   Decide what you want to think about the situation. What are your beliefs about yourself and life that drive your thoughts (self-fulfilling prophecy)?
        Thoughts » Feelings » Behaviors/Actions

3.  Choose the behavior.
    •   Decide how you are going to handle the situation.

Identifying **escalating behaviors** in a client early on can prevent the situation from getting out of control:

• Angry facial gestures
• Anxiety
• Breathing changes
• Demanding behavior
• Destruction of property
• Distended neck veins
• Furrowed brow, forceful words and/or tone of voice (cursing out loud)
• Hands clenching and unclenching
• Hand wringing
• Teeth clenching
• Increased voice, tone
• Mumbling to self
• Red face
• Refusing medications
• Standing in corner or closed area
• Verbal threats to peers and staff
• Large motor activity:
  • Pacing
  • Pounding hand into the other hand
  • Swinging arms

Aggressive behavior may be precipitated by:

• Trying to protect a vital interest
• Alcohol, drug abuse
• An aggressive or hostile staff member

- Change in role identity
- Expectation of staff
- Illness
- Lack of alternative methods of expression
- Lack of individual space
- Loss of freedom and self-direction
- Loss of meaningful activity and sense of purpose
- Mental illness/mental retardation
- Physical disabilities
- Physical pain

The following nursing interventions can be performed to prevent escalating behavior/situations:

- *Milieu Management:* Reduce/eliminate environmental/external stimuli. Decrease lighting/noise. Encourage patient to use relaxation techniques in room.
- Use affective involvement WITH OPTIONS.
  - For example, "Things feel tense. Should we discuss it now, or after there is some cooling-off time?"
  - Identify issues leading to the difficult/aggressive behavior when possible.
  - Exploration and understanding are the first phases of the helping process—not problem solving.
  - Encourage verbalization of fears/anger/anxiety instead of action on feelings.
  - Encourage deep breathing exercises if client is open to this.
  - Use positive expectations rather than negative consequences.
  - Speak slowly and softly, in a calming manner, even if the patient does not immediately respond. Less is more.
  - Approach an aggressive patient as if you expect the patient to be in control.
  - Maintain eye contact
  - Give the patient the choice of controlling the behavior or having staff help to control the behavior.
  - Indicate it is best for the patient remain in control.

*Figure 4-1. Assault Cycle*

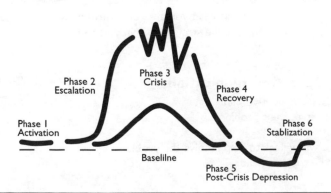

If the client's behavior continues to escalate despite verbal interventions, medication may be offered as an alternative intervention if ordered and appropriate.

- If ordered, provide PRN medication if patient's behavior continues to escalate.
- Oral medication is preferred during Phase 1 (activation) and Phase 2 (escalation) of the assault cycle (See Figure 4-1); however, if patient escalates into phase 3, IM medication will be required.
- If patient is psychotic, Haldol or Zyprexa can be helpful.
- PRNs are very helpful (e.g., Haldol, PO vs. IM; use IM if the patient requires more expedient intervention to de-escalate the behavior).
- If patient is not psychotic, PRN Ativan (short half-life) can be helpful.
- Depakote is often used to stabilize mood and will decrease and often eliminate physical outbursts.

*Remember, patient safety is the priority goal!*

## Communication Skills When Working with a Difficult or Aggressive Client/Individual

- Express caring and empathy: "Because I am concerned about your well-being, I want you to know I am available to speak with you about what you are feeling."
- Check out "whys" of behavior. Ask: "What is going on that causes you to be so upset?"
- Check out nonverbal messages. State, "I notice that you are wringing your hands and you are pacing down the hallway. Tell me how you are feeling."
- Use "I" statements. State, "I am concerned about your safety and the safety of others right now, as you are swearing and yelling loudly. I need for you to quiet down."
- Own your own feelings.
- Criticize the behavior, not the individual: "I want you to know that I care about your and others' health on this unit, however, your behavior of yelling and stomping around the unit is not acceptable."
- Positive stroking: find something genuinely positive to say, such as: "I admire how you were able to calm down after your father came to visit. I am confident you can calm down today as well."
- Point out what is in it for the patient: "When you are able to calm down and talk to me in a calm, respectable manner, I will sit down and talk to you about _____."
- Balancing message: "I know that what you are going through is very difficult for you, however, I know that you have the strength within you to cope in a manner that will help you in the long run."

## Rules for Open Communication
*Collaboration equals cooperation.*
- Both parties state their problem.
  - Use "I" statements.
  - Indicate a willingness to help resolve the problem.
  - Stick to the topic at hand.

- Hear them out.
  - Acknowledge the fact that you know they are angry.
  - Don't interrupt unless they are repeating themselves, then re-phrase what was said.
  - Acknowledge their viewpoints.
  - Ask clarifying questions.
  - Use silence.
  - Rehearse.
- Look for areas of agreement.
  - Point out general interests (why they want it) that you have in common.
  - Make an optimistic statement.
- Request behavior changes only.
- Help individuals help themselves.

## Changing Difficult Behavior

Nurses can do much to influence the individuals around them. Before labeling someone's behavior as "difficult" it is only fair to be sure you have done your best. If difficult individuals are treated with respect, they will respond differently and probably will not be so difficult anymore. Oftentimes difficult individuals usually think the other individual is the one who is being difficult. When asked to explain their difficult behavior, difficult individuals usually say they are acting in response to the other individual; if the other individual changes, the difficult individual will no longer believe they have reason to be difficult.

# Seclusion and Restraint

The nurse will provide the least restrictive environment for each client. However, if the patient's behavior continues to endanger self and/or others, the RN will need to obtain a specific order for restraints/seclusion from the attending or coordinating physician. The order includes a description of the criteria in which the restraint/seclusion may be applied and criteria for its discontinuation.

## General Principles

- A restraint is a device that will prevent the patient from moving at will and is applied to protect the patient from harming self and/or others.
- A patient may be placed in a locked seclusion room for aggressive behavior to protect the patient and others from the aggressive behavior of the patient.
- In an emergency, if a physician cannot be reached the RN may initiate and order the procedure and contact the MD as soon as possible.
- The procedure/policy for seclusion/restraint will vary from state to state.
- The RN will need to obtain an MD order within 1(one) hour upon initiation of the restraint/seclusion.
- Restrain only if other less restrictive measures have been tried without success.

Reassess the patient every 4 hours for purposes of determining continuation or release of restraints. It is absolutely necessary for all restrained patients to be offered the following every 2 hours:

- Offer and assist with food at meal and snack times or more often as indicated.
- Assist in hygiene, bathroom, use of urinal, commode, bedpan; offer fluids at least every 2 hours while patient is awake.
- Release restrained limbs and provide ROM exercises every 2 hours during waking hours and as needed during the night.
- The RN needs to provide assessment for trial release from restraints at least every 4 hours.

# Suicide

## Understanding Suicide

Suicide is a major complication of depression. Fifty to 70% of suicides in the US are due to depression. About 15% of severely depressed individuals commit suicide. In one study, the number of suicides among patients with mood disorders was about 80 times higher than in the general population and 8 times higher than in those with other psychiatric disorders. In the US, the risk of suicide is highest in older adult white males and in those who live alone, have made prior suicide attempts, refuse psychiatric evaluation, or abuse alcohol or drugs.

Risk factors for suicide include:
- Previous suicide attempt
- Mental disorders, especially mood disorders such as depression and bipolar disorder.
- Dual disorders (i.e,. mental disorder along with alcohol and/or substance abuse).
- Family history of suicide.
- Hopelessness.
- Impulsive and/or aggressive tendencies.
- Barriers to accessing mental health care and treatment.
- Relational, social, financial or work loss.
- Physical illness.
- Influence of important individuals (e.g., family members, peers, celebrities who have died by suicide; influence due to direct individual contact or inappropriate representations by the media).
- Cultural and religious beliefs (i.e,. believing that suicide is a noble act or an acceptable resolution of a individual difficulty).
- Epidemics of suicide (locally) can have a contagious influence.
- Isolation, a feeling of being cut off from other individuals.

(U.S. Public Health Service [1999]. The Surgeon General's Call to Action to prevent suicide. Washington, D.C.)

## Major Contributing Demographic Characteristics

Not to be included in the ratings, but considered in the overall assessment of suicide risk:
- Male (especially older, white male).
- Living alone.

- Single, divorced, separated, or widowed.
- Unemployed.
- Chronic financial difficulties.

Protective factors against suicide (U.S. Public Health Service, 1999):
- Appropriate and effective clinical care for mental, physical, and substance abuse disorders.
- Easy access to a variety of clinical interventions and support for seeking help.
- Restricted access to highly lethal methods of suicide.
- Family and community support.
- Ongoing supportive relationships in medical and mental health care.
- Learned life skills in conflict resolution, problem solving, and nonviolent handling of disputes.
- Cultural and religious beliefs that support self-preservation and discourage suicide.

Early warning signs of suicidal behavior:
- Suicide talk or threats.
- Giving away prized possessions.
- Withdrawal from significant others.
- Sudden changes in mood.
- Loss of self-worth.
- Loss of interest in individual appearance.
- Failure in school or poor job performance.
- Hypochondria
- Increase in substance abuse.
- A preoccupation with death.

## Critical Item Suicide Potential Assessment
*Primary Risk Factors*
**Attempt** (If ANY ONE factor is present, obtain consultation from psychiatrist or from another health care practitioner)

- Suicide attempt with lethal method (firearms, hanging/strangulation, jumping from high places).
- Suicide attempt resulting in moderate to severe lesions/toxicity.
- Suicide attempt with low rescue-ability (no known communication regarding the attempt, discovery unlikely because of chosen location and timing, no one nearby or in contact, active precaution to prevent discover).
- Suicide attempt with subsequent expressed regret that it was not completed AND continued expressed desire to commit suicide OR unwillingness to accept treatment.

**Intent**
- Suicidal intent to commit suicide imminently.
- Suicidal intent with a lethal method selected and readily available.
- Suicidal intent AND preparations made for death (writing a testament or a suicide note, giving away possessions, making certain business or insurance arrangements).
- Suicidal intent with time and place planned AND foreseeable opportunity to commit suicide.
- Suicidal intent without ambivalence or ability to see alternatives to suicide.

• Presence of acute command hallucinations to kill self whether or not there is expressed suicidal intent.
• Suicidal intent with CURRENT ACTIVE psychosis, especially major affective disorder or schizophrenia.
• Suicidal intent or other objective indicator of elevated suicide risk but mental condition or lack of cooperation preclude adequate assessment.

### Secondary Risk Factors

The following factors all significantly contribute to suicide risk, but are of a less critical nature. For the purpose of this instrument, all factors are considered of equal importance. (Obtain consultation from psychiatrist or another staff member if, in addition to some indication of increased risk, seven out of thirteen factors are present).

• Recent separation or divorce.
• Recent death of significant other.
• Recent loss of job or severe financial setback.
• Other significant loss/stress/life changes interpreted by client as aggravating (victimization, threat of criminal prosecution, unwanted pregnancy, discovery of severe illness, etc.).
• Social isolation.
• Current or past major mental illness.
• Current or past chemical dependency/abuse.
• History of suicide attempt(s).
• History of family suicide (includes recent suicide by close friend).
• Current or past difficulties with impulse control or antisocial behavior.
• Significant depression (whether clinically diagnosable or not), especially if accompanied by guilt, worthlessness, or helplessness.
• Expressed hopelessness.
• Rigidity (difficulty with adaptation to life changes).

This assessment tool was adapted from the Critical Item Suicide Potential Assessment from Hennepin County Medical Center, Minneapolis, MN 55415.

## Myths about Suicide

*Fable:* Individuals who talk about suicide do not commit suicide.

*Fact:* Of any ten individuals who will commit suicide, eight have given definite warnings of their suicide.

*Fable:* Suicide happens without warning.

*Fact:* Studies reveal that the suicidal individual gives many clues and warnings regarding his/her suicidal intentions.

*Fable:* Improvements following a suicidal crisis means that the risk is over.

*Fact:* Most suicides occur within about three months following the beginning of "improvement," when the individual has the energy to put his/her morbid thoughts and feelings into action.

*Fable:* Suicide strikes much more often among the rich, or conversely, it occurs almost exclusively among the poor.

*Fact:* Suicide is neither the rich man's disease nor the poor man's curse. Suicide is represented proportionately among all levels of society.

*Fable:* Suicidal individuals are fully intent on dying.

*Fact:* Most suicidal individuals are undecided about living or dying, and they "gamble with death," leaving it to others to save them. Almost no one commits suicide without letting others know how he/she is feeling.

*Fable:* Once a individual is suicidal, he/she is suicidal forever.

*Fact:* Individuals who wish to kill themselves are suicidal only for a limited time period.

*Fable:* Suicide is inherited or "runs in the family."

*Fact:* It follows individual patterns.

*Fable:* All suicidal individuals are mentally ill, and suicide is always the act of a psychotic individual.

*Fact:* Studies of hundreds of genuine suicide notes indicate that although the suicide individual is extremely unhappy, he/she is not necessarily mentally ill.

## Treatment for Suicide Prevention

Methods of handling the suicidal individual:

- Take suicidal threats seriously and evaluate the risk.
- Help individual identify a safety network (e.g., friends, family, church, neighbor, coworker).
- Remove all lethal objects.
- Ask about suicidal plan and intent.

Acute possiblity of suicidal behavior:
- Hospitalization of the client for stabilization.

No imminent risk for suicide:
- Create a therapeutic alliance with the patient.
- Psychiatric assessment/medication management.
- Exploration of feelings (i.e,. sadness, resentment, guilt).
- Group therapy.
- Use of cognitive-behavioral techniques.
  - Cognitive techniques:
    - Assist patient in identifying options and alternatives.
    - Thought-stopping techniques.
    - Encourage cognitive dissonance.
  - Behavioral techniques (examples):
    - Activity scheduling.
    - Social skills/assertiveness training.
    - Bibliotherapy (short readings).
    - Relaxation, medication, breathing.

## Aftercare Recommendations

- Relapse Prevention: Assist patient in identifying triggers and warning signs.
- Assist client in identifying support from others (i.e,. friends, family, support groups, mental health professionals, clergy).

# Caring for Patients, Families, and Caregivers Affected by HIV and AIDS

Since HIV is more common among homosexual and drug users, the patient with HIV or AIDS often has the two-fold problem of being judged for his lifestyle and for his disease. He needs compassion and understanding. It is important to take an inventory of one's biases. The gay men's population in the United States totals more than 12 million. The nurse/therapist's role is not only to counsel the patient, but also the family, friends, and caregivers. This is a challenge indeed.

## Human Immunodeficiency Virus (HIV)

The human immunodeficiency virus is a protein capsule containing ribonucleic acid (RNA). In normal body cells, RNA is synthesized from DNA (deoxyribonucleic acid) to carry the information needed for the development of an organism. HIV is called a "retrovirus" because its genetic information passes in the reverse direction, from RNA to DNA.

### Diagnosis

Being HIV positive means that the patient has human immunovirus in his system. The Enzyme-linked Immunosorbent Assay (ELISA) is a test that can determine whether a sample of blood serum contains antibodies to HIV. Also known as the enzyme immunoassay test, it can indicate, by the presence of the antibodies, if the individual is infected with HIV. There is a window period for HIV infection. By approximately 6 months after exposure to HIV, the patient tests positive. Therefore, a patient in a high-risk category should be tested every 6 months.

The diagnosis of AIDS is not made until the patient has had opportunistic infections. This can occur up to 10 years after infection, even without treatment of the virus. Opportunistic infections include toxoplasmosis, fungal diseases, cryptococcosis, and candidiasis. Non-Hodgkin's lymphoma and the viral diseases leukoencephalopathy and cytomegalovirus can attack the brain in AIDS. The T4 lymphocytes are the most affected cells in the immune system. They coordinate the responses of the immune system to biological invaders. The Center for Disease Control and prevention recommends a diagnosis of AIDS when the T4 concentration falls to 20% of normal. A significant loss of CD4 lymphocytes can indicate that the immune system is fighting AIDS.

### Mode of Transmission

In 2001, 16,000 individuals worldwide become infected with HIV each day. Until the introduction of antiviral drugs, almost all infected individuals developed AIDS. HIV is transmitted in three principal ways: 1) sexual activity; 2) contact with infected blood, primarily during IV drug use; and 3) HIV-infected pregnant women transmitting the virus to their babies before or during birth.

### Incidence and High-Risk Populations

AIDS is not a discriminatory disease. It strikes anyone. All nurses will encounter the disease. Sometimes they will be aware of it. At other times they will not be aware of their patient's infection.

HIV infection is most common among **gay men** and IV **drug addicts** in the US. The homosexual who practices unsafe sex and who uses drugs has an increased potential for infection. HIV infection in women is growing at a higher rate than it is growing among men in the United States. In the United States HIV is more likely to occur among women of color. HIV is the leading cause of death among **African American women** in the 25–44-year-old age group. It is the third leading cause of death among Hispanic women in the same age group. In 1996, white women accounted for 21% of all AIDS cases in women. Hispanic women accounted for 19%, and Afro-American women accounted for 59%. Women are often diagnosed later in their disease. Women have less access than men to routine and state-of-the art HIV/AIDS care. There are fewer support groups organized for women with HIV disease. Women often neglect their own health to take care of others. Many learn of their own HIV status only after giving birth to a child who later develops AIDS.

**Africa** accounts for two-thirds of the estimated 40 million HIV-infected individuals in the world. More than one in three adults who live in Botswana or Zimbabwe are infected with HIV.

From 1983 to 1989, the age of death for all **hemophiliacs** in the United States dropped from 63 to 38 years. The death rate due to AIDS rose in them from 20% in 1983–85 to 55% in 1987–89. Since 1985, heat treatment has been used in the preparation of clotting factors to inactivate HIV and eliminate this cause of HIV transmission. As of early 1997, the National Hemophilia Foundation knew of no new cases of HIV infection due to contaminated clotting factors since heat treatment began.

Individuals suffering from **chronic mental illness** are another group with high vulnerability to HIV and AIDS. They are all too often living on the streets, sexually active, and possibly using IV drugs. Education and testing is important in this population.

## Medical Treatment of HIV/AIDS

Many anti-HIV drugs became available in the United States in the late 1990s. In 1997, the year after the advent of the powerful drug cocktails, the U.S. death rate from AIDS dropped by 42%. The decline reflects improvements in medical care, better use of prophylaxis, and treatment for opportunistic infections. In 1998, the drop was only 20%. The number of new AIDS cases has nearly doubled from 1997. A true cure is still elusive. A vaccine is the best hope. Research is promising that HIV disease will become medically manageable and will be considered a chronic rather than a terminal disease in most cases.

To make DNA from its RNA, the virus uses the enzyme reverse transcriptase. Azidothymidine (AZT) was the first drug used to cripple this enzyme. Other reverse transcriptase inhibitors have been introduced. Protease inhibitors can reduce the amount of virus in the blood by 99% and raise the T4 cell count to nearly normal. Patients taking a combination of reverse transcriptase and protease inhibitors and other antiretroviral drugs can live for many years. Patients must continuously take several pills a day at carefully timed intervals to keep their immune systems functioning properly. Patients have their immune system monitored regularly through CD4 lymphocyte counts. They often also receive appropriate prophylaxis for Pneumocystis carinii pneumonia (PCP).

## AIDS Dementia Complex (ADC)

Confusion, apathy, and dexterity problems may emerge before more classic AIDS symptoms become apparent. It is unclear how exactly the human immunodeficiency virus (HIV) causes early neuropsychological symptoms, but studies do show that HIV can infect cells in the nervous system directly. The most common direct central nervous system complication appears to be a degenerative brain disease dubbed AIDS dementia complex (ADC). Its earliest signs can mimic depression with symptoms of hopelessness, insomnia, forgetfulness, poor concentration, and mental slowing. The Centers for Disease Control has revised its definition of AIDS. Only a positive HIV-antibody test, with or without signs of immunosuppression, would be required if the patient has mental symptoms associated with ADC. Many AIDS-related psychiatric problems are directly linked to the virus. These routes to infection contrast with the brain damage due to later opportunistic infections among immunosuppressed individuals. These patients now qualify for government disability benefits. Neurological and psychological tests may help detect evidence of HIV brain infection prior to clinical signs. Infected white cells (macrophages) localize quickly in the brain. They may release toxic substances that impair brain function. The virus may also damage the spinal cord and peripheral nerves. Loss of motor coordination is common. Tremors and paralysis may occur in the late stages. Poor judgment and socially inappropriate behavior are not uncommon. Ultimately, patients can become disoriented and even comatose. Anyone working with a high-risk group (homosexual, bisexual or IV drug users) should be alert to behavioral changes and mental symptoms. If psychotic symptoms occur, neuroleptic medication may be indicated. Antidepressants are sometimes advisable.

Communication with an individual with severe AIDS dementia complex can be difficult, as with any patient with dementia. Ask simple questions and respond to questions with simple answers. Long-term memory is often more intact. Ask about early experiences. Immediate memory may be severely impaired. Discuss home safety with the caregiver. Suggest arranging furniture to minimize risk of injury while maximizing freedom of movement. Keep the living areas brightly lit and move unstable furniture to reduce the risk of falls. Have calendars and clocks displayed to help keep the individual oriented as to date and time. Keep dangerous objects stored safely.

## Counseling the Patient with HIV/AIDS

### Pretest Counseling
When a patient asks for an HIV test, his counseling should start right away. Pretest counseling provides information about HIV disease, including its transmission and prevention. It also provides information about all sexually transmitted diseases. Signed informed consent is obtained for the testing and blood is drawn. The patient will return to learn about the test results. Always refer to the illness as HIV unless the patient has progressed to an actual diagnosis of AIDS (Ward, 1999).

### Post-Test Counseling
If the test is negative, the nurse discusses the importance of safe sex and avoiding other risky behaviors. Reinforcement of the information taught can be done. Individuals at high risk should be informed not to donate blood. If the individual remains at risk, recommend that he return for retesting at appropriate intervals.

If the patient is HIV positive, he needs counseling on several fronts. He needs help to avoid being in denial about his diagnosis. He should be encouraged to take advantage of early anti-HIV therapies and of preventive treatment of opportunistic infections to ensure a longer survival rate from the illness. He needs emotional and psychological support. Help the individual work through his feelings about the positive test result. Provide the names of physicians with experience in treating individuals infected with HIV. Discuss who should be told about the individual's HIV-positive status. Provide written information on individualal care, HIV disease, and preventing transmission of the virus to others. Refer the individual to the health department or local AIDS service organization for help in locating needed resources.

*Available Resources*
- The AmFAR AIDS Handbook (1999) by the American Foundation for AIDS Research and Darrell Ward is available in public libraries across the country.
- The National AIDS Hotline operated by the Center for Disease Control and Prevention (CDC) is an important source of HIV information. The toll-free number is 1-800-342-2437. The national hotline can also provide your state's HIV/AIDS hotline number.
- Local AIDS service organizations have information on local support groups, financial, legal, and social services, and state HIV drug assistance programs. They can also provide the names of the local physicians who are experienced in treating individuals with HIV disease.

*Legal Issues*
Several legal issues arise from HIV/AIDS. Confidentiality of the patient vs. rights of the caretakers to know the patients HIV status is a complicated issue. Rules about reportability of the illness to public health institutions have been changed and interpreted different ways in different states. There has been discussion of applying the Tarasoff law in the case of intentional infliction of the disease. Medical record confidentiality and negligence due to improperly informing an individual of exposure to HIV are important. Become familiar with your local state and agency regulations regarding these issues.

*Therapeutic Concerns*
Ideally the individual dealing with the spectrum of HIV/AIDS illnesses would receive group support and individual counseling to address the multitude of issues he or she must struggle with. Often this extensive care is precluded for a variety of reasons. Screen for concomitant depression in this population and treat appropriately. Encourage individual therapy. Clinical nurse specialists and psychiatric nurse practitioners often are the ones doing this therapy.

Group therapy provides support for patients who are amenable to it. Often these groups are comprised of patients who have been abandoned by friends and family because of their lifestyles. Denial, guilt, shame, and social stigmatization are problems they sometimes face. Issues of facing a potentially fatal disease must be faced. In most communities, there are agencies that provide such needed support.

## Support of Significant Others
The partners, significant others, and family members have special needs. If the patient is homosexual, the family may not be aware of it or may have withdrawn support. The partner of the patient is the primary support. One study found that in 25% of gay couples, the uninfected partner was more anxious and depressed than the one with HIV (Harvard Mental Health Letter, 1999). Also, some homosexual couples both have the disease or the patient you are seeing has lost his partner to the illness. Finding out who the patient's supports are is critical. Frequently the patient with AIDS will dwell on his own relationship with his family of origin.

## Nurses' Responses

Fear and misinformation can interfere with nursing care of patients with HIV/AIDS. Healthcare workers are at risk for infection in certain situations. If the attitude communicated by the nurse in a leadership position is positive to the patient with AIDS, many things can happen. In an informal study done in San Francisco, special qualities, desirable attitudes, skills, and attributes deemed most important in working with the patients with AIDS were compiled and listed in order of importance.

* Emotional stability.
* Enthusiasm and a sense of humor.
* Exceptional patience, understanding, and tact.
* A capacity for accepting differences and the ways in which affection or hostility may be expressed.
* A willingness to do custodial tasks, such as feeding, lifting, toileting, and handling of wheelchairs, beds, and cots.

As the leader of patient care, the nurse is in the position to set the climate in the environment to give support and acceptance to the patients with AIDS. Burnout is frequently the reason nurses leave an AIDS unit. Support for the caregiver is essential. The team approach, in which all the caregivers are working together for the welfare of the patient with AIDS, is most effective. Burnout is not experienced as quickly in the team approach. Nurses who work with patients with AIDS must have realistic estimates of their own strengths and weaknesses. They need sufficient security to accept these limitations comfortably. Nurses must examine their feeling about dealing with terminally ill patients.

## Issues of Death and Dying

AIDS is a potentially fatal disease. Individuals tend to die as they have lived. "Death is terrible to Cicero, desirable to Cato, and indifferent to Socrates." Dying as a psychological event is more elusive than the physical death. The fear of death has been broken down into the specific fears of pain, loneliness, abandonment, mutilation, and fear of loss of self. Death anxiety is a factor in caring for the AIDS patient. Studies agree that aging and illnesses alone do not necessarily cause death anxiety. Death anxiety is associated with anxiety and maladjustment in general.

Elisabeth Kubler-Ross (1969) is well known for her work with terminally ill patients. Her book *Death and Dying* is the classic work in thanatology. She and her associates interviewed hundreds of dying patients aged 16–96 years. Almost all socioeconomic levels were represented. The majority of them were from Judeo-Christian backgrounds. Muslims, Hindus, and atheists were included. Despite differences in cultural or religious backgrounds, the terminally ill patients did not vary in their basic needs. Their rituals sometimes differed.

Dr. Kubler-Ross divided the pattern of behavior of dying patients into five distinctive stages. These phases do not necessarily follow in the same order and a patient can move back and forth between them throughout the course of the illness. The first stage is shock and disbelief. The second stage is anger. The patient releases his anger in many directions and forms. He may be angry at the doctors and nurses and with relatives and friends. He may be angry with God. The third stage is bargaining. He may bargain with God for time. The fourth stage is reasonable depression. Sometimes this is called anticipatory grief. The final stage in the process of death and dying is acceptance. This phase is not always reached. The anxiety level declines to a moderate range. This is the time that patients put their world in order. They make their wills. Understanding does not always equal acceptance. A patient and family can understand that the prognosis is bleak, but not be ready emotionally to accept the information. With assistance, patients and loved ones can reach acceptance.

In 1987 Kubler-Ross published *AIDS: The Ultimate Challenge*. She discusses the problems encountered by the babies who were infected with HIV at birth. She writes of the partners of heterosexuals and bisexuals who have been infected. She examines the problems of those infected through blood transfusions, including hemophiliacs. The ethical balance between public health regulation and individual privacy is also discussed.

## Summary

Caring for individuals with HIV and AIDS is a challenging and rewarding experience for any nurse. It requires a multitude of skills and special individual qualities. Special sensitivity to the special needs of this population is involved.

# Alternative, Complimentary, and Expressive Therapies: Art, Music, Play, Dance, and Relaxation

Human beings are infinitely complex; therefore, the treatment of individuals with emotional problems and psychiatric illnesses is multifaceted. In approaching our patients as bio-psycho-social-spiritual beings, we must be open to whatever helps to heal that individual. The alternative, complimentary, and expressive therapies of music, play, art, dance, and relaxation can at times augment more traditional approaches to treatment. They can be effective ways to connect with a patient and heal a patient when other approaches fail or cannot be used. A child who cannot speak may be approached with art, music, or dance in addition to play therapy. An individual in a psychotic state can often be helped with relaxation techniques or music until the psychosis can be controlled. Anxiety disorders are immensely aided by teaching the patient relaxation techniques and by using art, play, music, and dance to relieve anxious feelings. All of these forms of therapy work by stimulating the senses. There are special training programs in these types of therapeutic interventions. Adaptability, flexibility, sensitivity, regard for human dignity, a sense of humor, and knowledge of therapeutic needs are all essential components of individuals working with complimentary and expressive therapies in the clinical setting.

## Art Therapy

Art therapy utilizes an individual's artwork as a means of communication and expression, rather than relying primarily on verbalization to understand the individual. The artistic creations can contain clues or insights into the individuality of the individual. It is the process and the content of the art produced that is important, not the end product. Art therapy can be appropriate for a wide range of individuals, from sophisticated adults to nonverbal, developmentally delayed children to psychotic patients. It provides an acceptable and controlled outlet for emotions and conflicts that otherwise might remain unexpressed in verbal therapy. The expression of dreams, fantasies, and conflicts into images is encouraged. The goals of therapy can be ego strengthening, catharsis, uncovering emotions, developing impulse control, and developing an ability to integrate and relate.

During art therapy the patients is observed for facial expression, tension, and other general observations. The work that is done is observed for repetition, colors, size, and/or theme. These observations can then be used therapeutically.

## Music Therapy

Music therapy involves listening to music, playing in rhythmic bands, singing, moving to music for relaxation and enjoyment, and getting in touch with feelings evoked when different types of music are heard. Music crosses over many diverse barriers—intellectual, cultural, and linguistic. Rhythm is the energizer of music. Music integrates the left and right brain hemispheres. It operates at a subliminal level. It is capable of producing a trance- like state, which in turn promotes relaxation and the ability to focus. Music combined with guided imagery is very effective because it continues subliminally where the verbal message leaves off. Music has been used successfully as a distracter in dental patients and in those with chronic pain.

## Play Therapy

Play therapy utilizes a child's play as a medium of expression to enhance communication between the child and the therapist. Since playing is a natural childhood activity, it can help resolve issues through free expression and learning. Play provides a safe and natural environment for children to express themselves verbally or behaviorally. It also provides for the learning of social skills such as taking turns, working out problems, creating your own fun, and getting along with others. The therapist can also use play therapy to uncover clues to the root of the child's problem. Children repeat demonstrated aggressive and other dysfunctional behaviors. Play therapy is usually nondirective and observational.

## Relaxation Therapy

Relaxation therapy is teaching patients to relax using such techniques as deep breathing, muscle relaxation exercises, guided imagery, and visualizing about being in a favorite place. The goal is to decrease anxiety by inducing a state of relaxation. Relaxation therapy is often used in conjunction with music and art. It can be used in conjunction with behavioral therapies such as systematic desensitization and biofeedback. Many of these relaxation techniques are used for pain management and in childbirth.

## Dance Therapy

Dance therapy is another form of expressive therapy. It involves expressing feelings through the rhythmic body movements of dancing. Rigid, nonverbal, or repressed patients are sometimes able to express themselves through this medium what they cannot express in other ways. Done regularly, it can also be an aerobic exercise with all of the accompanying benefits that such exercise entails.

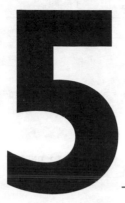

# Administration/ Management

## Outcome Evaluation

Outcome evaluation is a critical issue in the practice of APRNs, because managed behavioral health care has demanded that APRNs quantify outcomes of their practice and use outcome criteria to enhance the value of their clinical practice. This emphasis on outcomes provides an excellent opportunity for the APRN to document and provide evidenced-based information of the value of their contributions to psychiatric mental health care.

Definitions
* *Outcome:* "A measurable change in a client's health status related to the receipt of nursing care" (Marek, 1989).
* Outcomes are the results of interventions and treatments.
* Outcomes are the results received due to desirable and undesirable changes in an individual's or a population's health care that is attributed to the care that is provided (Donabedian, 1990).

Stuart (1998) identified four categories of outcome indicators or domains:
* *Clinical Outcome Indicators:* Coping responses. High-risk behaviors. Medical complications. Relapse. Readmission. Recurrence. Number of treatment episodes.
* *Functional Outcome Indicators:* Activities of daily living. Functional status. Social interaction. Family relationships.
* *Satisfaction Outcome Indicators:* Patient and family satisfaction with the caregiving process, health care delivery system, outcomes, and providers.
* *Financial Outcome Indicators:* Number of mental health care visits. Cost per treatment episode. Revenue per treatment episode.

## Quality Improvement

Definitions
* QC = Quality Control
* QA = Quality Assurance

- CQI = Continuous Quality Improvement
- QI = Quality Improvement
- TQM = Total Quality Management

Quality determination requires very specific measurable indicators and measurements/assessments of, if, or how well, the goal is being achieved.

### Reviews and Audits

*Nursing Audit:* The process of data collection and analysis. Data is related to nursing practice or patient outcomes. Analysis is used to evaluate the appropriateness or effectiveness of nursing care.

*Retrospective Audit:* A clinical study in which the patients or their records are investigated after they have experienced the disease or condition.

*Concurrent Audit:* A clinical study in which the patients or their records are investigated at the same time as they have experienced the disease or condition.

### Risk Management

Risk management refers to reducing one's liability in clinical practice. Ways of reducing one's liability in clinical practice include following protocols (e.g., dosing guidelines). Utilize nationally recognized guidelines that can serve as a basis for clinical pathways.

### Peer Review

Peer review is one type of performance appraisal/evaluation. Some common errors that can occur in a peer review evaluation:

- *Halo Effect:* The performance evaluation is positive due to the employee recently doing an outstanding job in caring for a client, despite poor work that was done previously all year long.
- *Horns Effect:* The performance review is negative due to recent poor performance on the job, despite excellent work that has been done all year long.
- Error of recency.
- *Contrast Error:* Contrasting with self or other individuals.
- *Central Tendency Error:* Tending to evaluate to the middle.
- *Error of Leniency:* The performance review was too easy on the employee.
- *Error of Severity:* The performance review was too harsh on the employee.

# Resource Utilization

## Access to Health Care

Many APRNs will be in situations where they will encounter underserved clients. Because of the impairment that can be caused by mental illness, the APRN needs to be alert to how clients have or do not have access to mental health care. It is necessary for the APRN to assist in protecting clients who are underserved and speaking up for these individuals, especially when judgment and reasoning are impaired due to their mental illness. Where a clinical practice is located is very important to the success of an APRNs practice.

The following elements are important when considering access to health care for your clients:
- Characteristics of the market that is being targeted.
- Location of the client's home and workplace.
- Length and mode of daily commute.
- Family status.
- Waiting space and office space image.

## Reimbursement

Reimbursement is an important issue, especially for the APRN in private practice. The price for service must be fair and consistent with the current rate within the community in which the APRN is practicing. The APRN can find out what is customary and can look for ways to add value to his or her practice (e.g., being readily available, immediate appointment scheduling, utilizing sliding scale fees based on income). The APRN may want to consider being a provider for as many third party payers as possible.

When setting up a practice, it can be helpful to send an application (each insurance company has its own application) to as many insurance companies as possible. When calling the insurance company, ask for "provider services." Ask them to send an application to be a mental health provider and to send their reimbursement payment scale. This will show the amount of money the insurance company is willing to pay the APRN for a variety of services (e.g., individual therapy, family therapy, group therapy).

Most insurance companies update their provider handbooks yearly and do so during the fall. Applying prior to the fall season can help a practice in being listed in the provider handbook at the next printing. Since most organizations are concerned with the amount of revenue that the APRN can generate, the APRN may want to consider creative ways of providing care, for example:

- Conducting groups (e.g., if $30 per group is charged per individual and there are 8 group members, $240 can be generated per group hour) in addition to providing individual therapy.

- Developing clinical pathways in collaboration with medical staff (e.g., when a client presents to the medical clinic for symptoms of hypothyroidism, the client can also be referred for mental health care if needed). This will increase the APRNs referral base.

## De-institutionalization and Community Mental Health Delivery

In the 1960s the concept that clients in mental institutions could be better served in the community was embraced and became public policy. Programs were designed using primary, secondary, and tertiary preventive care, yet these programs were based on the medical model within the framework of psychiatric pathology. The focus ultimately was on giving psychiatric clients medications to manage their illness, rather than on preventing hospitalization. In this movement, the psychiatric clients were "housed" and were not offered services where the clients would be taught life skills that would assist them in becoming productive members of society. The majority of individuals with mental illness live with family members or significant other(s).

Home care services have thus been necessary for those clients that are home bound and have an active psychiatric diagnosis. Medicare will pay for psychiatric home care if the client meets the following criteria:
• The client has been evaluated by a physician.
• A physician reevaluates the client every 60 days.
• The client requires skilled psychiatric nursing interventions by a psychiatric nurse.
• The client is home bound.

(Krainovich-Miller & Rosedale, 1999)

Such skilled psychiatric nursing interventions that can be provided in the home include:
• Conducting a comprehensive assessment.
• Performing venipunctures for liver function monitoring or medication monitoring.
• Providing psychoeducation.
• Providing psychotherapy.

(Krainovich-Miller & Rosedale, 1999)

## Policy and Program Development

### Definitions
• *Policy:* Goal or intended course of action.
• *Procedure:* A statement of technique to be followed when performing a given task.
• *Protocol:* Technique for a more detailed or complex procedure.
• *Case Management:* A health care delivery process with goals of quality care, decreased fragmentation of services, and cost containment.

### Local, State, and Federal Regulations and Guidelines
Policy involves "the application of reason, conscious decision-making, and problem-solving" (Haber & Streff, 1999). "Policy includes a broad range of activities that involve the establishment of authoritative guidelines in the form of laws or other official rules and regulations, position statements, or documents that deal with an issue of public concern and affect the conduct of public affairs" (Haber & Streff, 1999).

Five common types of policy (Haber & Streff, 1999):
• *Public policy:* A policy that is formed by a governmental body such as the Congress.

• *Social policy:* Policies that promote the public welfare of a segment of the population.

• *Health policy:* Policies that promote the health of citizens within a community.

• *Institutional policy:* Policies that govern the workplace and assist in accomplishing its goals (e.g., the institution develops and implements a policy for clients who wish to file a grievance against a hospital employee. The policy would include the grievance process for reporting and handling this incident).

• *Organizational policy:* Rules that govern an organization and the positions taken by an organization (e.g., the American Nurses Association passes a policy that opposes a registered nurses' participation in assisted suicide; the policy supports and affirms the organization's values and beliefs).

## Collaboration in Health Policy Formulation

APRNs are involved most often in institutional policy and organizational policy. There are a variety of ways in which the APRN can become involved in changing health policy formulation, including having knowledge of the policy stakeholders, being in touch with elected or appointed officials, and recognizing and using power.

Power is "that which enables an individual to accomplish goals" (Haber & Streff, 1999). There are eight types of power that can assist the APRN in being an effective leader/administrator:
- *Referent:* Given to others by association with others.
- *Legitimate:* Received from an organizational position or title.
- *Coercive:* Depends on another's fear of punishment.
- *Reward:* Obtained from the ability to grant favors or reward others with whatever they value.
- *Expert:* Received from knowledge and skill.
- *Charismatic:* Received from the individual's characteristics that cause him or her to be well liked.
- *Information:* Results when one individual has the knowledge or skill that the other individual wants or desires.
- *Self:* Received due to maturity and ego strength.

## Development of Community Programs

Large amounts of time and energy are required to develop and initiate new community programs. For mobilization of community efforts to occur, the following components are necessary:
- motivation to participate;
- reward for participating;
- participant needs are congruent with the outcomes;
- involvement in groups; and
- commitment and dedication.

There is an emphasis on community involvement rather than community participation. The former is more consistent activity, whereas the latter is variable (Meleis, 1992).

To develop a successful community program, it is necessary to conduct a community needs assessment.

# Leadership

## Definitions
- *Leadership* is defined as the ability to set and influence the direction of others: the dynamic interaction between leaders and followers.
- Leadership entails building a vision, trust, and commitment in interpersonal relationships.
- Leadership involves empowering others. It is concerned with creating a vision, shared goals, values, and commitment.
- Leaders influence behavior.

## Effective leaders:
- unite, motivate, and turn groups into teams;
- inspire and develop individuals and teams; and
- cooperate and collaborate with others.

## Staff Assignment

Barter and Furmidge (1998) defined assignment as the transfer of the activity or task and the accountability for the outcome. Parts of the assignment may be transferred from a registered nurse to an assistant (who is certified or licensed to complete the task or activity). This process is called delegation. The nursing care delivery system or structure of a particular nursing unit is the process that assists in guiding how assignments and delegated activities occur.

## The Decision-Making Model

- The NCSBN (1995) provides a model for the delegation decision-making process. The model follows the nursing process. The decision-making model includes:
  - Assessment:
    - Delegation criteria
      - Review qualifications of delegate
      - Review qualifications of delegatee
      - Delegation appropriateness under the nurse practice act.
    - Situational assessment
      - Assess needs of patient
      - Assess care setting
      - Assess available resources
  - Planning
    - Plan the tasks involved
      - Ascertain the implications and effect the delegation has for the patient and others.
      - Identify the task(s) to be performed and knowledge/skills that are required to perform the task/activity.
      - Demonstrate and document current competence of the delegatee for each task.
    - Plan for accountability
      - Assure that the delegator has accepted accountability for the performance of each tasks and activity.
      - Assure that the delegatee has accepted accountability for the proper performance of each task and activity.
    - Implementation
      - Direct the task performance and clearly state or document the expectations to the delegatee.
      - Monitor the delegatee's performance and assure that the policies, procedures, and standards of practice are followed properly. Intervene if necessary.
      - Document properly all tasks performed.

- Evaluation
  - After the completion of the delegated activities/task, evaluate the patient.
  - Evaluate the performance of the delegatee.
  - Provide feedback to the delegatee.
  - Review the care plan and modify as needed.

## Staff Conflict and Morale

The issues of staff conflict and morale are extremely important for the APRN to consider, especially given the fact that the morale of the staff or a conflict between staff members on a given unit will directly affect patient care (parallel process). Thus the APRN needs to be observant and proactive if and when low to moderate morale is demonstrated on the part of employees, or if staff conflict is ensuing on the unit. Low to moderate morale is easily recognizable as demonstrated by the following behaviors:

- frequent employee call-ins
- no shows
- quarreling among staff
- apathy
- complaints from patients regarding attitudes of the nursing staff
- work slowdown
- negative conversational tone while staff is in shift report or on breaks
- frequent staff turnover

Generally, when a staff member is having difficulty with another staff member and it is brought to the attention of the nursing supervisor, it is best if the nursing supervisor encourage the staff members to work the issue(s) out for themselves. The nursing supervisor can act as a sounding board or as a means to assist in facilitating resolution of the issue(s). The staff members can be encouraged to follow the problem-solving strategies covered in the crisis intervention section of this study module and the strategies for problem solving listed below.

## Staff Supervision

NCSBN (1990) states that supervision in nursing is defined as a qualified nurse who provides initial direction, guidance, and periodic inspection of a nursing activity or task and assures the task's accomplishment. ANA (1993) reports that supervision is an active process, including directing, influencing, and guiding the outcome of an individual's performance of an activity/task. The supervision can take place either on-site or off-site. Other duties that may be entailed in the role of providing staff supervision, including: 30, 60, 90 day performance reviews for new employees, setting of professional goals for the next 12 months, annual performance reviews, hiring, performance improvement plans for employees, providing and/or guiding the training of new employees, and recruiting.

## Innovative Problem Solving

The steps of the problem-solving process include:
- Gather information regarding the problem.
- Define the problem
- Develop solutions. If an individual is part of the problem, he or she can also be a part of the solution. Include the individual for brainstorming about possible solutions.

- Consider the consequences for each alternative solution.
- Make a decision.
- Implement and evaluate the solution.

(Huber, 2000)

*Strategies for Problem Solving (Huber, 2000)*
- *Direct intervention:* This strategy entails personally taking action. It is carried out by direct physical or verbal activity to intervene in a situation and to resolve a problem.
- *Indirect intervention:* The nurse manager/supervisor may use his/her interpersonal communications skills to work around the problem. Conflict resolution, confrontation, negotiation, and persuasion are examples of indirect intervention.
- *Delegation:* Assign a specific task or activity to a qualified individual.
- *Purposeful inaction:* A conscious decision is made to not act or do anything about the problem. The premise behind purposeful inaction is that with time, the problem will go away.
- *Consultation or collaboration:* Exchanging ideas and information with a peer. This strategy is related to coordinating and networking with others.

## Consensus Building

Consensus building or joint decision making is an approach where the entire group decides either by two-thirds vote, a simple majority, or a consensus. In this situation, the subordinates have as much power in the decision-making process as the leader. Generally, when consensus is utilized as the decision-making process, the subordinates will feel more a part of the team. The CNS leader can use the following actions to assist in building consensus:

- Enable group members to participate in the decision.
- Communicate vision and enthusiasm for group goals.
- Motivate followers to accomplish group goals.
- Model positive group participation.
- Inspire team collaboration.
- Facilitate and model constructive group roles.
- Monitor the process of the group.

(Huber, 2000)

# section two

## Child and Adolescent Psychiatric-Mental Health Nursing

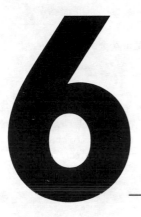

# History, Practice and Legal and Social/ Cultural Issues

### Parent's Creed   *by Kahlil Gibran*

"And a woman who held a babe against her bosom said: Speak to us of children. And he said: They are the sons and daughters of life's longing for itself. They come through you but not from you, and though they are with you, they belong not to you. You may give them your life but not your thoughts, for they have their own thoughts. You may house their bodies but not their souls, for their souls dwell in the house of tomorrow, which you cannot visit, not even in your dreams. You may strive to be like them, but seek not to make them like you. For life goes not backward nor tarries with yesterday. You are the bows from which your children as living arrows are sent forth."

## Psychiatric Mental Health Nursing Practice

### Clinical Practice Settings
Nurses in child psychiatry may provide services to prenatal clinics, day care centers, nursery schools, and other child care programs where preventive care includes health education in the areas of infant and child development, child rearing and parenting. Counseling for life stressors such as divorce, death, or chronic illnesses can also be done. The clinical specialist may provide consultation to day care centers, nursery schools, and pediatric floors in the hospital.

### Interventions
Interventions may involve early diagnosis and treatment and prompt referral as necessary. Such a setting in child psychiatry might be in an outpatient clinic or a partial hospitalization program where the nurse would use a variety of modalities to help families cope during crises. The clinical specialist could be asked to consult with schools to provide coordination of services relative to a child experiencing emotional difficulties.

### Common Settings for the Clinical Specialist
Child psychiatric inpatient unit of a general hospital and transitional care settings such as day care, group homes, and outpatient clinics where the nurse serves predominately as a

milieu therapist, helping the child deal with daily life occurrences; and providing a healthy adult-to-child relationship and role model.

## Summary

The clinical specialist can work in organized health care and be salaried, contracted, or receiving fee for service. Self-employment is another option: the clinical specialist can have a solo or group practice that provides services to EAPs, HMOs, PPOs, managed care companies, industrial health departments, home health agencies, and nurse-owned businesses.

## Legal Issues in Treating Minors

*Definition of a minor:* Individual under 18, unless emancipated.

*Emancipated minor:* At least 14 and legally married or in the military or has filed a petition of emancipation with the court which states that he is 14, managing his own financial affairs with no illegal income, and willfully living away from the parents and with their consent. NOTE: Petition won't be granted if court determines that emancipation would not be in minor's best interest.

*Confidentiality:* The minor has the same rights as an adult. An emancipated minor is legally an adult. At the beginning of treatment this should be with the minor and the parents, defining what information will be shared and what will be private.

*Privilege:* Confidentiality relating to legal matters; parents usually hold the privilege to disclose or not to disclose in a court of law.

*Exceptions to parents:* The therapist can refuse to allow parents to inspect the records when the minor is the victim of a crime; when there is a court-appointed guardian/custodian holding privilege; when a therapist is seeing the minor without parental knowledge or consent; and when the therapist asserts the privilege for the minor.

*No parental consent:* When the minor is 12 or older and provides good reason to not involve parents and is mature enough to participate intelligently in outpatient treatment. Clinical issues that can be treated with no parental consent include: when minor seeks help for substance abuse; when minor needs help with prevention or treatment of pregnancy; when child has been the alleged victim of incest or child abuse (including rape); and when minor might be a serious threat, mentally or physically, without treatment. Also, a minor can consent for treatment of infectious or contagious disease.

*Fees for treatment of a minor:* Parents are not held responsible for payment for treatment of their minor child when the parent has not been contacted and has not given consent. The minor can also authorize release of medical records.

*Therapist responsibility:* Involve parents in treatment of a minor unless the therapist believes it is not in the best interest of the minor. The therapist must chart in the record if or when the parents were notified or, if not notified, why it was considered inappropriate to do so.

*Exceptions to minor's giving consent:* Minors are not authorized to sign for abortion, sterilization, psychotropic drugs, methadone treatment, convulsive therapy, or psychosurgery.

## Custody

*Joint custody:* Term meaning joint physical custody and joint legal custody.

*Sole physical custody:* A child shall reside with and under the supervision of one parent, subject to the court's power to order visitation.

*Joint physical custody:* Each of the parents will have significant periods of physical custody that will be shared by the parents to assure a child of frequent and continuing contact with both parents.

*Sole legal custody:* One parent will have the right and responsibility to make the decisions relating to the health, education, and welfare of the child.

*Joint legal custody:* Both parents have the right and responsibility to make the decisions relating to the health, education, and welfare of the child.

# The Law and Juveniles

All fifty of the United States have juvenile court laws, but the first juvenile court as we know it today was established in Cook County, Chicago, Illinois.

Minors are defined as all individuals under the age of 18 years. The authority of a parent ceases:
• Upon the appointment by a court of a guardian of the minor
• Upon the marriage of the minor, or
• Upon attaining majority (18)
• Upon the process of the "Emancipation of Minors Act"
  • One who has entered into a valid marriage, or
  • One who is on active duty in the US military, or
  • One who has received a declaration of emancipation

The purpose of the emancipation for the minor is:
• For consenting to medical, dental, or psychiatric care, without parental consent, knowledge, or liability.

• For the purpose of the minor's capacity to: enter into a binding contract, buy, sell, lease, trade, exchange real property, sue or be sued in his/her own name, compromise, settle, arbitrate, or adjust a claim, action, or proceeding by or against the minor, make or revoke a will, make a gift outright or in trust, create a revocable or irrevocable trust, revoke a trust, renounce or disclaim any interest acquired by testate or interstate succession.

NOTE: Laws may differ from state to state. The above laws apply to California. There are a few more, but this gives you a good sample.

# Cultural Issues

## Native Americans
• Link state of health to good or evil forces.
• May view illness as punishment.

- Use spiritual rights, homemade remedies, mechanical devices.
- Strongly independent, reluctant to accept help.
- Elders are respected as leaders, teachers, and advisors.
- Greet both men and women with a soft handshake.

## Black Americans
- May have health problems related to lower standard of living.
- May hold unconventional beliefs.
- Look to family for decision making.
- May feel cautious as a defense against prejudice.
- Have higher levels of self-esteem.
- Are less likely to receive prescribed stimulants than are Caucasians.
- Avoidance of eye contact is a self-protective adaptational stance.
- Frequently over-represented in the diagnosis of disruptive behavior.

## Jewish Americans
- Strong sense of identity and shared beliefs.
- Religious traditions are important to most Jews.
- Saturdays are their Sabbath; may oppose procedures on Saturdays.
- May cling to belief that head and feet should always be covered.
- Orthodox Jews may oppose shaving.
- Kosher diet is significant.
- Support modern medicine but may want rabbinical consultation on major decisions.
- Family bonds are very strong.
- Autopsies are usually opposed.

## Chinese Americans
- Believe in yin (female negative energy) and yang (male positive energy).
- May prefer traditional treatments to modern medicine (e.g., acupuncture).
- Compliant nature; may not express discomfort or disagreement easily.
- High regard for older adults, families care for their own.
- Avoidance of eye contact as sign of respect.

## Japanese Americans
- Generally more integrated into American society than the Chinese, but many still cling to tradition.
- Compliant natures similar to Chinese.
- Family unit is strong; older adults are viewed with respect.

## Hispanic Americans
- Many feel states of health are acts of God.
- Medals and crosses may be worn at all times to facilitate well-being.
- Prayer plays an important part in the healing process.
- Illness may be viewed as a family affair with multiple members involved.
- Some may prefer traditional practitioners to modern medical services.
- Elders are held in high esteem.
- Males expect firm handshake; females expect a soft handshake.

## Summary

- Caregivers should be aware of language differences and realize that stress of illness may decrease the patient's ability to communicate in English as a second language.

- Consult with patient and/or family members regarding traditions of their culture. Showing an interest in their culture sends a message of sensitivity and caring.

# History of Child Psychology

## Definition

Child psychology includes the study of the child's heredity, physical constitution (biological, chemical, and physiological processes), and the environmental forces to which he or she is exposed. All of these, working together, affect physical and intellectual growth, psychological health, and social adjustment. The process of personality development is continuous starting from conception, and involves the interaction of a biological organism with its physical, psychological, and social environment, all of which are functionally related to each other.

## History

Writers throughout history have shown interest in child psychology. Plato recognized the importance of early childhood training in determining later vocational aptitudes. In his *Republic,* he discussed differences between children and recommended taking steps to assess aptitudes and to provide education and training at an early age to coincide with a child's particular strengths and talents.

In the seventeenth century, John Locke published an essay, "Some Thoughts about Education," which maintained that infants' minds are blank tablets at birth and are receptive to all kinds of learning. Locke said that the object of all education is self-discipline, self-control, and the power of denying ourselves the satisfaction of our own desires, where reason doesn't authorize them. "From their cradles" children were to begin instruction in self-denial. Locke's ideas are similar to the "formal education" of today.

In the late eighteenth century, French philosopher Jean Jacques Rousseau believed that the child is born with an innate moral sense, intuitively knowing right from wrong. He believed that restrictions placed on children by adult society thwart children and force them to become less virtuous. In *Emile* he wrote of the child as a "noble savage." Rousseau advocated a back-to-nature movement that would encourage inherently noble impulses. His philosophy influenced the progressive schools' stressing spontaneity and freedom of expression. As in modern psychological thinking, he believed that individual development is influenced mostly by the experiences of the first years of life.

In 1774, a Swiss named Pestalozzi published notes based on observations of his 42-month-old son's development. In 1787, Tiedemann published a book on the infant during the first 27 months, tracing sensory, language, motor, and intellectual growth. In the nineteenth century, many "baby biographies" began to appear; they usually were accounts by the babies' own relatives. One of these biographies was by famous biologist Charles Darwin; another was by Bronson Alcott, father of Louisa May Alcott, author of *Little Women.* Those kinds of biographies, although interesting, were usually biased, positive, unsystematic, and contained observations made at irregular intervals. However, they did have some value and contained many hypotheses about the nature of development.

Toward the end of the nineteenth century, Dr. Stanley Hall, a US pioneer and president of Clarke University who was interested in studying the contents of children's minds, began a systematic study of larger groups of children. He devised a new research technique, the questionnaire, which aimed at obtaining information about child and adolescent behavior, attitudes, and interests. He collected written responses to questionnaires from both children and parents. His research continued into the twentieth century and was the beginning of systematic child study in the US. Hall's research wasn't controlled or highly objective, but he did use large numbers of subjects to get representative data and tried to determine the relationship between background experiences, adjustment problems, and personality.

In the early 1900s, child psychiatry began developing from four major bodies of knowledge: education, psychology, psychoanalysis, and information obtained from working with delinquent youth. Sigmund Freud recognized that early childhood experiences played a major role in the mental health of the adult and developed a technique called "analysis." Two analysts working in the 1920s and 1930s, Melanie Klein in Berlin and Anna Freud in Vienna, played major roles in the development of psychoanalysis. Klein used play therapy as the key to treating mentally disturbed children, while Freud's major emphasis was on developing a positive transference with her patient through playing with toys. Later they continued their work in the US and in England.

Through their normative studies, Binet, Catell, and Gisell developed the concept of intelligence and laid the cornerstone for Erikson's developmental theory, which was further studied by Dewey and James, two educational psychologists who were wondering how a child learns. Their work brought knowledge from education to psychology for application in the teaching and testing of children. Pavlov, Watson, and Skinner, who described stimulus-response learning, established the behaviorist school of thought. Jean Piaget, a Swiss psychologist, advanced the developmental theory of cognitive growth; he called the school-age years the concrete operations stage and noted that they mark the beginning of the age of reason.

During the Industrial Revolution in the United States, the great flux of immigrants caused an increase in juvenile delinquents and homeless orphans. Foster homes were established in the early 1900s. W. Healy studied delinquency in Chicago and concluded that many things caused delinquency, not the least of which was the role of the family. The child guidance movement began in the 1930s and the court system initiated the psychiatric treatment of children, which later became community based.

Nurses were initially custodial caretakers in the field of psychiatry until the advent of somatic therapies between 1930 and 1940, when it was felt that some effort should be placed on educating nurses in psychiatry to give better care to psychiatric patients. The National Mental Health Act of 1946 provided funding for advanced training of psychiatric nurses and other professionals in undergraduate and graduate nursing programs. In the next decade Boston University established a graduate program for child psychiatric nurses.

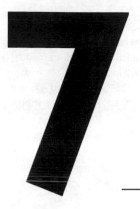

# Developmental Disorders

## Mental Retardation

### Definition

"Mental retardation refers to significantly sub-average general intelligence functioning resulting in or associated with impairments in adaptive behavior and manifested during the developmental period" (American Association of Mental Deficiency, and recently, by the American Psychiatric Association). For many years, adaptive behavior has been ignored in the definition, but now it has to be looked at in terms of community responsibility for the individual and others. The DSM-IV-TR further clarifies that the onset must be prior to age 18.

General intellectual functioning is defined by the intelligent quotient (IQ or IQ equivalent) obtained by assessment with one or more of the standardized, individually administered intelligence tests such as the WISC-III, which evaluates the present level of intellectual functioning, the Stanford Binet Intelligence Scale-Fourth Edition, and the Kaufman Assessment Battery for Children.

The latest in the field of assessments are the behavioral assessment, which describes human responses that are controlled by environmental events, and the focal assessment, which is specific to narrower areas of pathology and has a major advantage because of its efficiency, cost effectiveness, and evaluation of treatment modality. Technological advances in psychological testing, interpreting, and scoring by computer programs offer more sophistication, accessibility, and affordability.

### Degree of Severity

*Mild:* IQ from 50 to 55 to approximately 70. This group is usually educable to the second to fifth grade functional level.

*Moderate:* IQ from 35 to 55, trainable to live semi-independently.

*Severe:* IQ from 20 to 40. Cannot develop independent living skills. Usually due to biological causes.

*Profound:* Less than 20 to 25. Dependent on others for self-care-institutionalized. Biological causes.

NOTE: In assessment of severity, DSM-IV TR provides a separate code for Mental Retardation, Severity Unspecified, when there is a strong presumption but the individual is not testable by standard tests. The largest proportion of retarded individuals falls within the mildly retarded range (89%). In the moderate range, about 7%; between 3 and 4% are in the severe and profound levels. According to estimates, from 1% to 3% of the general population are mentally retarded.

## Epidemiology

More retardation than giftedness is indicated by the IQ distribution.
Two separate groups make up the retarded:
• genetically and environmentally predisposed, and
• prenatal or otherwise brain-damaged.

Numbers in the general population may change with age, depending on different definitions of adaptation.

Retardation is 1.5 times more common in males than in females.

## History of Mental Retardation

Around 1500 B.C. documents from Egypt were written that described mind and body disabilities and the brain being affected. In ancient Greece and Rome, it was common to practice infanticide if appointed examiners found a child defective. This practice diminished gradually during the middle ages (476-1799 A.D.) when John Locke, in 1690, had the belief that the mind was a blank slate. He also was the first to write about the difference between mental retardation and mental illness. In 1800, a physician named Jean-Itard developed a broad educational program to help children develop their senses, intellect, and emotions. His work was continued by another man named Edouard Seguin who developed an approach that began with sensory training of children with mental retardation. This was known as the Physiological Method. In 1876, he founded what today is the American Association of Mental Retardation. We still use some of his techniques today.

By 1908, Binet's intelligence test was translated by Henry Goddard, a researcher from Vineland, New Jersey's Residential Training School. These residential schools were established in many states for individuals who had mental retardation, and it was thought that these patients could be trained appropriately. In 1916, L.M. Terman classified the severity of symptoms of mental retardation with labels such as borderline for a 70-79 IQ, moron 50-69 IQ, imbecile 25-49 IQ and idiot with an IQ of 24 or below. It wasn't until 1961 that those labels disappeared on classification of severity. In 1935 Edgar Doll, who later in 1941 stated that mental subnormality is of "constitutional origin" and is "essentially incurable," developed the Vineland Social Maturity Scale. His discussion of constitutionality centers on the idea of biological pathology as the cause of mental deficiency.

As time went on, more residential schools were opened for the growing number of diagnosed mentally retarded individuals who, it was believed, could be cured with the right training. When the "cure" didn't happen, the schools became more custodial centers for the mentally retarded. Between the 1950's and the 1970's the National Association of Retarded Citizens and the President's Commission on Mental Retardation were established. In the 1970's, the Wyatt-Stickney federal court class action suit was filed in Alabama and gave the right to treatment to those retarded individuals living in residential facilities. In 1976, the US Congress passed the Education Act for the Handicapped (now known as the Individuals with Disabilities Act), which guarantees education for all children with developmental disabilities and mental retardation from school age to age 21.

In 1992, the American Association on Mental Retardation adopted the definition that "mental retardation refers to substantial limitations in present functioning and is characterized by significantly sub-average intellectual functioning, existing concurrently with related limitations in two or more of the following applicable adaptive skill areas: communication, self-care, home living, social/interpersonal skills, use of community resources, self direction, health and safety, functional academic skills, leisure and work. Mental retardation manifests before age 18.

## Trisomy 21 (Down Syndrome)

Down syndrome (DS) is a combination of birth defects including some degree of mental retardation and characteristic facial features; about 30-50% of individuals with DS also have congenital heart defects. Many have visual and hearing impairment and other health problems that vary greatly in severity. This is the most common genetic cause of developmental disability that we know of, and it affects all races and socioeconomic levels equally. DS is sometimes referred to as "mongolism." For many years we have known that the incidence increases in babies born to mothers over 35 years old. Some hereditary factors may increase the risk, and in recent studies, it is indicated that very young parents below 15 years of age are also at risk.

An English physician named J. Langdow Down first described the condition in 1866; it was the first autosomal genetic abnormality to be described in humans. It took until the 1950s for researchers to discover that, instead of 23 pairs of chromosomes (normal), individuals with Down syndrome have one extra chromosome with one of the pairs—thus the name trisomy 21. Almost all individuals with DS have this trisomy, but about 4% have an abnormality called translocation, in which a piece of one chromosome in the 21 pair breaks off and attaches itself to another chromosome.

Characteristics of the Down syndrome include several of the following: broad, flat face; upslanted eyes, sometimes with an inner epicanthal (mongolian) fold; low-set ears; small nose and enlarged tongue and lips; sloping underchin; moderate to severe retardation; heart or kidney malformations or both; and abnormal dermal ridge pattern on fingers, palms, and soles. Life expectancy among adults is about 55 years at the maximum, but there are exceptions.

## Pervasive Developmental Disorders (PDDs)

These disorders are characterized by severe and pervasive impairment in several areas of development: reciprocal social interaction skills, acquisition and use of language, and in leisure and play activities. There is no evidence that psychological factors cause these disorders.

### Autistic Disorder

*Definition:* A child is diagnosed as having an autistic disorder if he or she has a pattern of atypical development in the three areas of social skills, communication, and behavior. Most of these children are mentally retarded but differ from other mentally retarded in the development of those three areas. The autistic disorders are the most studied of all the

PDDs. The IQ level of affected individuals is usually between 35 and 50. Onset is during infancy or childhood and typically appears by the age of 3. These children have a remarkably restricted repertoire of activities and interest. They need things to stay constant—unchanging. The current generally accepted view that a set of recognizable behaviors constitutes a clinical syndrome of early childhood autism is based on Leo Kanner's work in 1943. The points he considered important to making a diagnosis were:

• A profound lack of affective contact with other people.

• An anxiously obsessive desire for the preservation of sameness.

• A fascination for objects, which are handled with skill in fine motor movements.

• Autism, or a kind of language that doesn't seem to be intended to serve interpersonal communication.

• The retention of an intelligent and pensive physiognomy of good cognitive potential, manifested in those who can speak by feats of memory and, in the mute children, by their skill on performance tests.

The Autism Society of America defines autism to be a complex developmental disability that typically appears during the first three years of life. The result of a neurological disorder that affects the functioning of the brain, autism and its associated behaviors have been estimated to occur in as many as 2 to 6 in 1,000 individuals (Centers for Disease Control and Prevention 2001). In this disorder there are impairments in social interaction, communication, and imaginative play prior to 3 years. Stereotyped behaviors, interest and activities are also symptoms.

Kanner also emphasized that the behavior pattern was present from early childhood. Later writers feel that autism and the other PDDs are complex neurodevelopmental disorders that usually appear during the first 3 years of life. Autism and related PDDs occur in approximately 15 in 10,000 live births and affect all races, cultures, and social groups. Some autistic babies are extremely placid and rarely cry or demand any attention. Others are restless, scream for long periods, and cannot be comforted. Disturbed sleep, erratic patterns of sleep, and feeding patterns including sucking are common. Later, prolonged rocking and head banging may be noticed. The children may show little interest in the human voice and lack interest in social contact. According to the DSM-IV TR, at least six of the following 12 descriptors must be present for a diagnosis of autistic disorder. At least 2 items from (1), one item from (2), and one item from (3):

1) Qualitative impairment in reciprocal social interaction as manifested by:

• Marked impairment in the use of nonverbal behaviors

• Failure to develop peer relationships appropriate to developmental level

• Lack of spontaneous seeking to share enjoyment, interest, or achievements with others

• Lack of social or emotional activity

2) Qualitative impairment in communication

• Delay in, or total lack of, the development of spoken language

• Marked impairment in the ability to initiate or sustain a conversation in individuals with adequate speech

• Stereotypical or repetitive use of language or ideosyncratic language

• Lack of various, spontaneous, make-believe play or social imitative play appropriate to developmental level

3) Restrictive repetitive and stereotyped patterns of behavior, interests, and activities

- Encompassing preoccupation with one or more stereotyped and restricted patterns of interest that is abnormal in intensity or focus
- Apparently inflexible adherence to specific, nonfunctional routines or rituals
- Stereotyped or repetitive motor mannerisms
- Persistent preoccupation with parts or objects

4) Delays or abnormal functioning in social interaction, language as used in social communication, or symbolic and imaginative play prior to 3 years of age

5) The disturbance is not better accounted for by Rett's disorder or childhood disintegrative disorder

Autistic children have inappropriate emotional variations. They don't have much understanding of other individuals' feelings. Inappropriate laughing, crying, and screaming can occur. One of the major problems with autistic children is the lack of imaginative play. Toys aren't used as material for imaginative games. Instead, the children tend to handle, taste, smell, and gaze at toys and other objects to experience simple sensations. Often they select minor or trivial aspects of objects or individuals to focus their attention on, such as a wheel instead of the whole toy train. The autistic child is intensely resistant to change and has attachments to objects and routines, which become very important to some of these children.

The classically autistic child has some areas in which he performs well, specifically, in the non-language-dependent skills such as fitting jigsaw pieces together, and secondly, in the skills relying on exact memory such as words to songs and poems. Memory for visual patterns also tends to be excellent. Problems occur in motor imitation—young autistic children find it very difficult to learn by watching and imitating. Language is another area where autistic children have problems. Their use of speech is abnormal. The control of vocal pitch, volume, and intonation is very poor, and unlike deaf children and those with developmental speech disorders, they do not gesture to compensate for their speech problems. They have poor compensation and use any form of language and nonverbal methods of communicating. Abnormalities of posture are sometimes present, as well. Examples include: walking on tiptoes, odd hand movements, and odd body posturing. Autistic children appear to have difficulty making use of incoming information from their senses. Variable response to sound is common, and they may be fascinated by some sounds while being distressed by others.

The physical characteristics observed most are the whirling and rocking of the body, which may be the child's way of making sense out of the environment, including his own body and its parts, through psychomotor feedback. When the body whirls, it tends to induce labyrinth stimulation in the middle ear; for some unknown reason, the autistic disordered child who whirls does not appear to get vertigo or dizziness, which leads to one theory that autism is caused by an organic defect in the left temporal lobe of the brain. Many cases of this disorder are associated with perinatal pathology of types known to lead to brain damage. Another theory is that there is possibility a genetic influence (2% of siblings of autistic children suffer from the same condition; this is 50 times that of the general population). Adults with autistic disorder do not tend to marry and reproduce. The fragile X chromosome is found in up to 16% of autistic males. In 1967 Dr. Bruno Bettleheim, a psychiatrist who ran a treatment program in Chicago for autistic children, described "refrigerator mothers" as contributing largely to autism. His idea had no supporting data.

A diagnosis of autism requires ruling out congenital disorders such as deafness, vision problems, retardation, speech problems, and other psychoses such as schizophrenia and fragile X syndrome. Appropriate psychological testing and a detailed study of the child's behavior patterns are necessary to ensure diagnostic accuracy, to assess the severity of the syndrome, to measure level of adaptive functioning in various domains, to test language and cognition (IQ), and to assure the validity of research findings. Some of the measures being used in Stanford University Hospital's Child and Adolescent Psychiatry Department's research include the Autism Diagnostic Observation Scale (ADOS), the Autism Diagnostic Interview (ADI), IQ tests (WAIS, WAIS-III, and WISC-III), the Vineland Adaptive Behavior Scale, the Peabody Picture Vocabulary Test, the Benton Facial Recognition Task, and the Judgement of Line Orientation task (JLO).

Currently there is no known drug that is effective in treating this disorder, but some drugs are effective in diminishing the symptoms displayed. Studies to evaluate medications such as risperidone (Risperdal) and valproic acid (Valproate) are investigating their effects on cognition, behavior, and development as well as their safety and efficacy. Evidence is emerging which suggests that certain genetic factors may confer susceptibility to this disorder. Some individuals with autism function at a relatively high level, with speech and intelligence intact, and others are developmentally delayed, mute, or have serious language difficulty. Much understanding and patience is necessary when working with these children as well as when educating and supporting their parents. In the home or school, the playroom needs to be very orderly and unchanging, with fewer toys and stimuli than would be in a normal playroom, and very safe. Favorite music, songs, poems, expressions, and objects will generally keep children with autism entertained. They seem to do better in a one-to-one relationship in a nonthreatening environment.

## Asperger Disorder

First described in the early 1940's by Hans Asperger, an Austrian Psychiatrist, who observed abnormal behavior in a group of adolescents and labeled them as autistic psychopaths. Meanwhile in the United States Leo Kanner was describing the same syndrome. Asperger syndrome or disorder is a particular type of pervasive developmental disorder that is characterized by problems in the development of social skills and behavior. In the past, many children with this disorder were diagnosed with autism, which has certain similarities to Asperger disorder. However, the differences are important, requiring careful evaluation before making the diagnosis.

The typical child with autism functions at a lower level than the child with Asperger disorder, who is typically of normal intelligence and is using words by the age of 2, although with somewhat odd speech patterns. Most children with Asperger disorder tend to be loners, having trouble interacting with their peers. Their behavior may appear to be eccentric. For example, they may spend hours preoccupied with counting passing cars on the street or watching just the financial channel on television. Difficulties in coordination are common because of clumsiness and they usually have special educational needs. Current research suggests that a tendency towards this condition may run in families, and children with this disorder are also at risk for depression, behavior difficulties, ADHD, schizophrenia, and obsessive-compulsive disorder.

The most effective treatment involves psychotherapy, special education, behavior modification, and support for families. Medication will benefit some with the disorder. The prognosis for children with Asperger disorder is better than for those with autism.

Because of their higher levels of intellectual functioning, many will finish high school and attend college. Even though they have problems with social interactions, they can have meaningful relationships with family and friends.

## Rett Syndrome

Rett syndrome is characterized by a severe impairment in expressive and receptive language development with severe psychomotor retardation. So far the syndrome has only been reported in females, and problems develop in coordination of gait or trunk movements. The child is normal during the first 5 months of life and then loses previously acquired hand skills. Her head growth decelerates between 5-48 months, resulting in microcephaly. Subsequently, characteristic stereotyped hand movements resembling handwashing or handwringing develop.

## PDD NOS

This is also a childhood disintegrative disorder in which the child develops normally until age 3-5, has better language and social skills than with autism, but doesn't meet the criteria for a specific pervasive developmental disorder.

## Childhood Disintegrative Disorder

The main characteristic of the disorder is a marked regression in multiple areas of functioning following a period of at least 2 years (and before 10 years) of apparently normal development of age-appropriate verbal and nonverbal communication, social relationships, play, and adaptive behavior. This condition has also been called Heller syndrome, dementia infantilis, or disintegrative psychosis. Children with this disorder have social and communicative deficits and behavioral features usually observed in autism.

## Fragile X Syndrome

Fragile X syndrome results from a chromosomal error in which the X chromosome breaks. The symptoms include poor eye contact, rapid or repetitive speech, and difficulty adjusting to change. An individual with the condition usually has mental retardation and distinctive characteristics such as prominent ears. The symptoms in males tend to be more severe than in females, and about 1 of every 2,500 females and 1 in 1,200 males will develop the disorder. Diagnosis is made by microscopic examination of the patient's chromosomes and analyzing the DNA.

# Learning Disorders

Learning disorders include: reading disorder, mathematics disorder, disorder of written expression, and learning disorder not otherwise specified (NOS). When the individual's achievement on individually administered standardized tests in reading, mathematics, or written expression is substantially below that expected for age, schooling, or level of intelligence, learning disorders are diagnosed. Approximately 5% of US public school students are diagnosed with learning disorders.

The school dropout rate for children and adolescents with learning disorders is reported to be at almost 40%. These disorders are found also in individuals with conduct disorders, oppositional defiant disorder, ADHD, and major depressive disorder or dysthymic disorder. The prevalence is 10–25%. From 60% to 80% of children with reading disorder are males. Mathematics disorder is seldom diagnosed before second grade and may not become apparent until fifth grade or later.

## Motor Skills Disorder

If there is a marked impairment in the development of motor coordination and it significantly interferes with academic achievement or activities of daily living, the diagnosis of Developmental Coordination Disorder is made, providing that the coordination difficulties are not due to a general medical condition and the criteria are not met for PDD. If mental retardation is present, the motor difficulties are in excess of those usually associated with it.

## Communication Disorders

Expressive language disorder, mixed receptive-expressive language disorder, phonological stuttering, and communication disorder NOS are all classified as communication disorders.

The most common expressive language disorder in younger children is **phonological disorder**, which is a failure to use developmentally expected speech sounds appropriate for the age and gender of the child. This involves failure to form speech sounds correctly—lisping is common. At least 2.5% of preschool children present with phonological disorders, which often are referred to as functional or developmental. When there is a disturbance in fluency and language formulation, **cluttering**—an abnormally rapid rate and erratic rhythm of speech and disturbances in language structure may occur. The developmental type of expressive language disorder is usually recognized by age 3. The acquired (functional) type due to strokes, brain lesions, head trauma, etc., will have sudden onset and occur at any age. An essential feature in **stuttering** is a disturbance in the normal fluency and time patterning of speech that is appropriate for the child's age. It may be accompanied by motor movements and can be brought on by stress or anxiety. Male to female ratio is 3:1. Onset is usually between 2 and 7 years old.

# Prenatal Factors Affecting the Newborn's Risk for Developmental Disability (See also Table 7-2)

## TORCH Infections (organisms crossing the placental barrier)

*Rubella (German measles).* It is in the first trimester before 10 weeks when most fetuses that are infected will get rubella. With cell division slowed by the disease, 50% of those infected will show slowed growth and fewer cells than normal. By age 5, 70% will show effects.

*Toxoplasmosis.* Due to primary maternal infection with the protozoa *Toxoplasmosis gondii,* which is found in many mammals, humans, and birds, toxoplasmosis can be treated to prevent further spreading in the body if it is detected (treated with Sulfadiazine and Daraprim). Mother and child are asymptomatic at birth. Of the infants infected, 15% will die and 85% will show severe psychomotor retardation. Today, women are screened for antibodies during the first prenatal visit.

*Hepatitis B.* Most infants are asymptomatic, but other disorders and prematurity or stillbirth can happen.

*Cytomegalovirus (CMV).* Most common cause of perinatal infection. CMV is a member of the herpes virus family and often causes no symptoms in the mother. The mother's infection can have occurred during this pregnancy or during a previous one; the virus can be dormant, and like herpes, reactivate. The baby can have birth deformities, seizure disorders, and blindness. Most problems show up when child is 3 to 7 years old and include lowered IQ, deafness, motor defects, and learning disabilities.

*Herpes virus (HV).* There is no definite link between herpes and any congenital disease, but when the mother has the primary genital herpes, prematurity, spontaneous abortion, and certain congenital anomalies can be associated. If the mother has open lesions in the birth canal and the infant is grossly contaminated, there is a 30-50% infection rate for infants by a vaginal delivery. Of those, 50% will die or have defects.

## Environmental Pollution and Drug Exposure

According to the American Chemical Society, there are over 110,000 different biologically active substances that may adversely affect the newborn's development by causing chromosomal abnormalities, nonchromosomal congenital abnormalities and defects, altered sex ratio, neonatal death, low birth weight, altered fertility pattern, spontaneous abortion, developmental disabilities, behavioral disorders, childhood malignancies, and childhood death.

- Macroenvironmental — from heavy metals, radiation, ozone, etc.
- Microenvironmental — (social environmental)
  - Tobacco smoke, carbon monoxide, nicotine, alcohol, polycyclic aromatic hydrocarbons. Adversely affect fetus by increased bleeding during pregnancy, long-term birth disorders, spontaneous abortion and rupture of the membranes.
  - Drugs — opiates, barbiturates, anesthetics, sex steroids, food additives—can produce developmental disabilities, congenital heart defects, etc., fetal death.

### Cocaine

Usually, the babies at risk are not identified until their mother goes into labor or when the newborn shows signs of stress at birth or shortly afterwards, as in the nursery. When examining the newborn, the alert nurse will look for a particularly small head circumference for gestational age, a regularly seen condition in cocaine-exposed neonates. Blood pressure may be elevated; changes in the EKG may be seen; necrotizing enterocolitis may occur, which will be suggested if there's abdominal distention, feeding intolerance, and vomiting.

Stool testing for occult blood should be done to confirm this condition. Infections, especially STDs (sexually transmitted diseases), should be evaluated and managed. Hepatitis B and HIV are highly possible and need to be managed also. If the maternal status is unknown and there are high risk factors such as IV drug use, HBIG (hepatitis B immune globulin) should be given immediately to the newborn.

The cocaine-exposed newborn is typically hypertonic when alert and can be easily overstimulated to the point of becoming irritable. However, when not alert, the newborn is lethargic and poorly responsive, tremulous, and disorganized in feeding and sleeping. Visual responsiveness is frequently not normal; nor is the auditory ability. Seizures occasionally occur by the second or third day of life (when the cocaine has probably cleared from the urine). Then, the most apparent neurobehavioral disturbances become apparent. Nurses can monitor neurobehavioral, autonomic and GI changes with the

Neonatal Abstinence Scale developed by Finnegan, which includes common signs of withdrawal such as hypertonia, jitteriness, hyperactive Moro reflex, tachypnea, loose stools, decreased sleep, excessive suck, nasal stuffiness, and poor feeding.

The certified clinical specialist in psychiatric and mental health nursing can be especially helpful when working with the parents of "cocaine babies" as well as with the nursing staff educating them about the psychological aspects of cocaine addiction, parenting of a hypertonic and irritable baby, the legal aspects of reporting antenatal drug exposure, managing the staff's negative and judgmental feelings about the mother's cocaine use, assessment and management of the care of the baby in the hospital, and planning for discharge and ongoing care. Staff and parents can be educated about finding resources available to support the mother and child in their rehabilitation. If the mother continues to use cocaine or other psychotropic drugs, breastfeeding is contraindicated.

### Fetal Alcohol Syndrome

When pregnant mothers drink excessive amounts of alcohol during their pregnancy, physical and mental defects may develop in the fetus. This combination of defects is known as FAS, or fetal alcohol syndrome, and is one of the most common known causes of birth defects producing mental retardation. It is the most common preventable cause.

The babies are unusually small at birth and don't usually catch up as they get older. Their eyes are usually small and widely spaced, and they have a short upturned nose and small flat cheek. They may suffer from a variety of organ malfunctions, especially of the heart. Most babies with FAS have small brains and are mentally retarded to some degree. Many are poorly coordinated, have short attention spans, and exhibit behavioral problems. Drinking during pregnancy can also increase the risk of miscarriages, stillbirth, and death in early infancy. Heavy drinkers are 2–4 times more likely to have a miscarriage between the fourth and sixth month of pregnancy than are nondrinkers. In the United States, one of every 750 newborns has FAS. That's about 5,000 babies per year—this compares to the number of children born with Down syndrome each year.

Women who drink 3 oz of pure alcohol each day frequently give birth to babies who have FAS. This amount of alcohol is the equivalence of 6 cans of beer or 6 mixed drinks or 6 4-ounce glasses of wine. Two to 5 drinks a day can also damage the fetus and produce some of the signs of FAS. These signs are called fetal alcohol effects (FAE). Some women can drink heavily throughout pregnancy and have children with NO signs of FAS. Alcohol passes through the placenta to the fetus soon after the mother drinks, and the baby gets the same amount as the mother, but the baby's organs are immature and do not break down the alcohol as quickly as in the mother, so the blood level of alcohol in the baby will be higher.

## Congenital AIDS

More than 75% of children who were born with AIDS had mothers who either had AIDS during pregnancy or belonged to one of the special risk groups. Many of these children became infected either before birth, while in the womb, or during delivery. A few have become infected later by breastfeeding. About 17% of children with AIDS received whole blood or blood products prior to early 1985 when the test to screen blood became available. Some children have become infected during sexual abuse.

Nurses, parents, and other caregivers who have close contact with AIDS-infected children or adults, such as sharing beds and eating utensils, are NOT at high risk for transmission of the AIDS virus. It is possible for a woman to be unaware that she has been infected by the virus until her infant develops AIDS. The infants who are infected with AIDS suffer frequent infections and diarrhea, and fail to thrive and gain weight. Enlarged lymph glands, spleen, liver, and salivary glands are common, and many children have delayed development, maybe due to brain damage from the virus.

The usual AIDS screening test, which detects blood antibodies elicited by HIV, is unreliable for an infant born to an infected mother, because if the baby has not yet been infected and HIV infection is suspected, an infant needs more definitive testing to prove the presence of HIV and to exclude other types of immune problems that are common in infants born to drug-abusing mothers. These immune problems usually occur in the first year of life and are NOT AIDS or an AIDS-related complex (ARC).

Infants with AIDS are closely monitored and treated with antibiotics, gamma globulin, or antiviral drugs when infections occur. NOTE: Live virus vaccines such as mumps, measles, and polio should NOT be given to a child infected with HIV or to other household contacts. The inactivated vaccine can be substituted for the live polio vaccine.

## Acquired Immune Deficiency Syndrome (AIDS)

AIDS is an infectious disease caused by the HIV virus, which attacks the white blood cells (T-lymphocytes) and the immune cells (CD4 cells)

HIV testing measures the number of antibodies that the body has developed in its attempt to fight the HIV virus. It takes 2 weeks to 3 months for the antibodies to show up in the HIV test. During this time, the individual can still transmit the virus to others.

*Transmission*
- Sexually transmitted
- Transmitted through blood contact or exchange
- Transmitted to newborns from an infected mother
- One out of 3 newborns born to infected mothers has AIDS

*Disease Process*
Three different responses to the AIDS virus:
- The individual may have no symptoms of illness and can still transmit the virus to others.

- Infected individuals may develop ARC and have symptoms less severe than those of classic AIDS, including loss of appetite, weight loss, fever, night sweats, diarrhea, skin rashes, tiredness, lack of resistance to infections, or swollen lymph nodes. These symptoms can be due to other diseases, so requires expert diagnostics to identify ARC.

- AIDS destroys the individual's immune system, making it vulnerable to "opportunistic infections" such as *pneumocystis carinii* pneumonia or Kaposi sarcoma.
  - "Opportunistic infections" take advantage of the compromised immune system of the AIDS patient. They would not otherwise be able to get a foothold.
  - "Opportunistic infections" are usually the cause of death for the AIDS patient.

*Treatment*
- Observation
- Clinical monitoring
- Primary care:
  - Nutrition
  - Health habits
  - Education
  - Support systems

Current therapies include anti-retroviral agents. There is no known cure or vaccine for AIDS at this time.

---

*Table 7-1. Typical Progression of Pathology by Age of Onset (read left to right)*

| Preschool | School Age | Adolescent |
|---|---|---|
| Developmental disorders age 2–3 Asperger's | Disruptive behavior disorder | Eating disorder Anorexia age 12–15 |
| Attachment disorder age 2–3 to 5–6 | Anxiety disorders | Bipolar |
| Neglect/abuse | Mood disorders such as Behavior disorder | Schizophrenia age 17 |
| Munchhausen by proxy | Tic disorders Somatoform disorders age 9 | Substance abuse Gender identity |
| Elimination disorders 1. Encopresis age 4 2. Enuresis age 5 | PTSD | Dissociative disorders |

---

# Developmental Disorders and the Newborn

The transitional period for the newborn is considered to be the first 24 hours of life. Adjustments need to be made during that crucial time—these include respiration, circulation, liver changes, kidney changes, and metabolism changes. Immediately after the delivery, the Apgar score is taken and recorded; in 5 minutes, the Apgar is repeated; within 6 hours after delivery the physiological status is assessed, as are the heart and respiratory rates and the gestational age. The next exam, a complete physical, is performed within 24 hours of life or when the infant is stable.

Five factors are included in the Apgar scoring: heart rate, respiratory effort, muscle tone, reflex irritability, and color. Each is rated with 0, 1, or 2 (0 indicating low or weak, 2 indicating high or strong), and the separate scores are totaled. Extremely low Apgar scores at 5-minutes suggest a potential problem. It has been noted that children with a 5-minute score of 3 or below have 3 times as many neurological problems at age 1 as babies of similar birth weights with Apgar scores of 7-10. Apgar scores of 6 or below are monitored carefully. Through biological-chemical analyses, newborn screening is further accomplished. Through analyses of blood specimens alone, there are 14 different inherited abnormalities that are detectable. They are (* = treatable):

- PKU (Phenylketonuria)*
- Emphysema (adult)*
- Maple syrup urine disease*
- Galactosemia transferase or kinase deficiency*
- Tyrosinemia *
- Hereditary angioneurotic edema
- Histidinemia*
- Orotic aciduria*
- Valinemia*
- Argininosuccinic aciduria*
- Galactosemia transferase deficiency*
- Liver disease (infant)
- Sickle cell anemia

*These disorders are treatable enough to diminish or prevent the developmental problem that would result if the condition was not known or was ignored.

---

Table 7-2. Effects of Commonly Abused Mood-Altering
Substances on Maternal, Fetal, Neonatal Well-Being

---

*Alcohol/Ethanol*

| | |
|---|---|
| Street names: | Suds, oil, short dog, short necks |
| Other: | Wine, beer, mixed drinks |
| In medicines: | Nyquil, Robitussin, Listerine, Geritol |
| Modes of use: | Drink |
| Maternal effect: | Acute withdrawal, sedation, inebriation, damage to organs (i.e., heart, liver, stomach) |
| Fetal effect by trimester: | *Throughout:* Fetal alcohol effects and fetal alcohol syndrome growth deficiency, microcephaly, stillbirth, decreased birth weight, joint and facial anomalies, genito-urinary anomalies, cardiac anomalies |
| In labor: | Acute withdrawal, transient muscular hypotonia |
| Neonatal effect: | Acute withdrawal with sedation, seizures, poor feeding |
| Developmental effect: | Developmental delay, hyperactivity, low IQ |

(Continued on next page)

## Table 7-2. Continued

### Amphetamines/Stimulants

| | |
|---|---|
| Names: | Crank, pinkhearts, crystal critters, Ritalin, pellets, pocket rockets, toot, go fast, go-go, blast, Adderall |
| Modes of use: | Snort, mainline, shoot drink, foil (heat and inhale vapors) pipes |
| Maternal effect: | Dilated pupils, euphoria, excitation, loss of appetite, increased blood pressure and heart rate, insomnia |
| Fetal effect by trimester: | *Throughout:* Intrauterine growth retardation (IUGR) *First:* bilary atresia, transposition of great vessels |
| Neonatal effect: | Tremors, hypertonicity, poor suck rate, and high-pitched cry |
| Developmental effect: | Long-term effects not known |

### Barbiturates

| | |
|---|---|
| Names: | Nembutal/pentobarbitol, Seconal/secobarbital, Phenobarbitol |
| Modes of use: | Oral |
| Maternal effect: | Habituation, sedation |
| Fetal effect by trimester: | *Delivery:* sedation |
| Neonatal effect: | Tremors, hypertonicity, poor suck rate, high-pitched cry |
| Developmental effect: | Long-term effects not known |

### Caffeine

| | |
|---|---|
| Names: | Brand names, No Doze tablets, cup of Java, coffee, tea, sodas |
| Modes of use: | Oral |
| Maternal effect: | Irritability, headaches |
| Fetal effect by trimester: | *Throughout:* Spontaneous abortion, stillbirth |
| Neonatal effect: | Decreased birth weight |
| Developmental effect: | Long-term effects not known |

### Cigarettes/Nicotine

| | |
|---|---|
| Names: | Smokes, cancer sticks |
| Modes of use: | Smoking, inhaling, patches |
| Maternal effect: | High tar and nicotine cigarettes cause some heart and lung problems |
| Fetal effect by trimester: | *Throughout:* Decreased birth weight and head size |
| Neonatal effect: | Jitteriness, poor feeding |
| Developmental effect: | Lower scholastic scores, increased rate of SIDS |

(Continued on next page)

## Table 7-2. Continued

### Cocaine

| | |
|---|---|
| Names: | Crack, goop, Hubbas, dove, medicine, chasing the dragon, rock, crystal, free base |
| Modes of use: | Smoke, snort, shoot, foil, heat and inhale vapors |
| Maternal effect: | Stimulation, tachycardia, hypertension, heart attacks |
| Fetal effect by trimester: | *First:* increased spontaneous abortion, congenital anomalies |
| | *Third:* abruptio placentae, cerebral infarction |
| Neonatal effect: | Tremors, hypertonicity, muscle weakness, seizures |
| Developmental effect: | Developmental delay, 4–15% increased rate of SIDS |

### Heroin

| | |
|---|---|
| Names: | Chasing the dragon, Chiva, China white, Mexican born, boy, hop, dog food, smack, Persian |
| Modes of use: | Outfits, mainline, snort, smoke, needles |
| Maternal effect: | Habituation, sedation |
| Fetal effect by trimester: | *Throughout:* Small for gestational age |
| Neonatal effect: | Withdrawal symptoms, tremors, hypertonicity, poor feeding, diarrhea, seizures, irritability |
| Developmental effect: | 5–10% increased rate of SIDS |

### Marijuana/Cannabis

| | |
|---|---|
| Names: | Pot, herb, smoke, residue |
| Modes of use: | Smoked |
| Maternal effect: | Sedation, hallucinations |
| Fetal effect by trimester: | *Prior to conception:* chromosome changes, decreased sperm counts |
| Delivery: | Bleeding problems |
| Neonatal effect: | Sedation, tremors, habituation, excessive response to light |
| Developmental effect: | Long-term effects not known |

### PCP/Phencyclidine

| | |
|---|---|
| Names: | Angel dust, KJ |
| Modes of use: | Smoked, injected |
| Maternal effect: | Hallucinations, agitation, nystagmus |
| Fetal effect by trimester: | *Delivery:* agitation |
| Neonatal effect: | Irritability, microcephaly at birth, uncoordinated fine motor skills, sensory input problems |
| Developmental effect: | Long-term effects not known |

## Evaluation Tools for Assessment of Intellectual Functioning in Young Children

The two classification systems being used today to diagnose and assess the disorders of the 0–3 year old are: the *Diagnostic and Statistical Manual of Mental Disorders, Fifth Edition* (DSM-IV-TR) and the *Diagnostic Classification of Mental Health and Developmental Disorders of Infancy and Early Childhood* (DC:0–3; Zero to Three, 1994). Some of the most common behavioral problems found in the birth to 3 years age group are: excessive crying, excessive fearfulness, feeding problems, separation/attachment difficulties, and sleeping problems. Each problem needs to be assessed to reach an appropriate diagnosis, and the DC:0–3 system is conceptually easier to understand than the DSM-IV-TR. For this reason, the DC:0–3 is beginning to be used in healthcare systems. The first three tests listed are designed to fit with the DC:0–3.

*The Infant-Toddler Social and Emotional Assessment (ITSEA)*
Uses symptoms that match the DC:0–3 and DSM-IV-TR diagnostic systems to diagnose infants and toddlers. This test was designed in 1999 by Carter, Little, Briggs-Gown, and Kogan. This test is a structured parental interview.

*Diagnostic Interview Schedule for Children (DISC)*
For children 3 to 8 years old, this is also a structured parental interview.

*Preschool Age Psychiatric Assessment (PAPA)*
This is an adaptation of the Child and Adolescent Psychiatric Assessment (CAPA) for children 2 to 5 years old. This, too, is a structured parent interview and is limited by its subjectiveness.

*Bayley Scale of Infant Development*
This test measures infant and toddler development from 1 to 42 months and has separate subscales for motor and mental performance. The test takes longer to administer.

*Child Behavioral Checklist*
One of the most widely used, this test measures children from 2 to 3 years based on reported behavioral problems as seen by parents.

*Vineland Adaptive Behavioral Scale*
This test measures the performance and ability of the child from 0 to 18 years in terms of progressing towards independence. Parents and teachers fill out this test.

*Parenting Stress Index*
This test measures the 0–10 year old according to parent's report of the parent-child system under stress.

*Infant and Toddler Mental Status Exam (ITMSE-1997)*
This is adapted from traditional mental status exam dimensions and includes new categories such as sensory response and self-regulations. Areas of functioning included in this assessment are appearance, motor, relatedness, play, self-regulation, affect and mood, thought, speech/language, and apparent reaction to situation.

*Revised Denver Developmental Screening Test*
This test is for children age 0–6 years and measures four areas of development: gross motor, fine motor, language, and personal-social; concentration of test items for birth to 18 months.

## Mental Status Exam of Children and Adolescents

In J. E. Simmons' book *Psychiatric Examination of Children*, the following areas are commonly covered in a mental status exam of children:

*Appearance*—description of the physical size, manner of dress, hygiene, posture, and any obvious handicaps

*Defense mechanisms*—description of major defenses the child uses to cope with anxiety

*Neuromusculature*—description of the child's ability to locomote in a coordinated fashion and to execute gross and fine motor movements

*Thought processes*—description of the child's thoughts (verbalized). Are they logical, cohesive, and secondary process, or are flights of ideas, loose associations, and primary process thoughts present? Is the child preoccupied or having hallucinations or delusions?

*Fantasy*—description of the child's ability to fantasize and know the limits of fantasy. This gives data about wish fulfillment, dreams.

*Concept of self*—description of the child's level of self-esteem, self-image, and self-ideal

*Orientation*—description of the child's concepts of time and ability to perceive who and where he is

*Superego*—description of the child's value system, ability to discern right from wrong, and ability to respond to limit setting

*Estimated IQ*—description of the child's general fund of information for his age and other age-appropriate tasks.

The mental status exam should take place in a relaxed environment without rush and stressors such as phone calls, interruptions, etc. Toys, games, dolls, cars, puppets, etc., should be visible and available in the exam room because their presence tends to lower the child's anxieties and are very useful during the assessment, particularly when verbal communication is difficult.

## Comparison of Developmental Theories

### Key Conflict

*Weaning (birth to 1 year)*
- Freud
  - Oral sensory stage substages
    - Passive
    - Aggressive
- Erikson
  - Basic trust vs. mistrust
- Piaget
  - Sensorimotor, sense of self, and object permanence

*Toilet training (1–3 years old)*
- Freud

- Anal stage substages
  - Retentive
  - Expulsive
- Erikson
  - Autonomy vs. Shame (age 2 years)
- Piaget
  - Beginning of symbolic play and language.
  - Characteristics:
    - Egocentrism
    - Magical thinking
    - Animism
    - Artificialism
    - Realism
    - Centration
    - Irreversibility
    - Preoperational period (ages 2–7)
      - Shows egocentrism and centering
      - Substages
        - Conceptual (age 1.5–4 years)
        - Intuitive (age 4–7 years)

*Oedipus and Electra complexes (age 3–6 years and age 5–9 years)*
- Freud
  - Phallic stage (age 4–6 years)
  - Beginning latency (age 7–12 years)
- Erikson
  - Initiative vs. guilt (age 3–5 years)
  - Mastery and industry vs. inferiority (age 6–12 years)
- Piaget
  - Enters stage of concrete operations (age 5–9 years)
  - Thought process based on a concrete point of reference rather than abstract

*Acquisition of cultural values (age 9–12 years)*
- Freud
  - Latency period ends (age 7–12 years)
- Erikson
  - Industry vs. inferiority continues
- Piaget
  - Stage of concrete operations continues

*Sexual expression (age 12–14 years)*
- Freud
  - Beginning stage of sexuality
  - Genital stage (age 12+ years)
- Erikson
  - Identity vs. role confusion (identity diffusion) (age 13-19 years)
  - May begin intimacy vs. isolation (ages 15-18 years)

- Piaget
  - Begins stage of formal operations (age 12+ years)
  - Reasoning about hypothetical situations-systematic search for hypothesis
  - Stage of formal operations (age 15-18 years)

---

## Table 7-3. Developmental Theory According to Erikson

*Synopsis of Erikson's Stages*

*Stage One*

| | |
|---|---|
| Age: birth to 1 year | Infancy |
| Physical involvement: | Sensory |
| Psychoanalytical terms: | **Oral** |
| Some radius: | Maternal |
| Attitudes and ego strengths: | *Task:* **Trust vs. mistrust, hope** |
| Emotional needs: | Security in being loved, fed, kept warm, etc. Consistency for predictable trust. Dependability of the feeding person to define one's identity as a separate person. |
| Frustrations: | Weaning |
| Personality characteristics and associated behavior: | Beginning ego development<br>• Sucking behavior<br>• Exploration of the body<br>• Rage reaction to frustration<br>• Crying, later biting<br>• Narcissism, passivity, dependency<br>• Low frustration tolerance |
| Mental Mechanisms and examples: | **Substitution** (displacement): thumb and nipple sucking activity |

---

*Stage Two*

| | |
|---|---|
| Age 1–3 years: | Toddler |
| Physical involvement: | Muscular |
| Psychoanalytical terms: | **Anal** |
| Some radius: | Parent |
| Attitudes and ego strengths: | *Task:* **Autonomy vs. shame and doubt, will, and purpose** |
| Emotional needs: | To make decisions, to learn control over body functions, to explore the physical world, to learn limits, to learn what is permissible; freedom from excessive shame and permission to express resentment. |
| Frustrations: | Development of sphincter control |
| Personality characteristics, associated behavior: | Beginning superego development, exploration of environment, smearing of feces, mud pie games, ambivalence, negativism, awareness of mother, father, siblings, sibling rivalry, and sex differences |

(Continued on next page)

## Table 7-3. Continued

| | |
|---|---|
| Mental mechanisms and examples: | **Introjection:** Standards of cleanliness and toilet training. **Projection:** Places blame for failure onto others. **Displacement (substitution):** Child becomes angry at parents, destroys toys, etc. |

### Stage Three

| | |
|---|---|
| Age: 3–6 years | Preschooler |
| Physical involvement: | Genital |
| Psychoanalytical terms: | **Phallic, Oedipal** |
| Some radius: | Basic family, siblings, playmates |
| Attitudes and ego strengths: | *Task:* **Initiative vs. guilt;** identification with sex |
| Emotional needs: | To test, to find out what's wrong, to learn control over body functions, to satisfy sexual curiosity, to differentiate reality from fantasy, to have adequate parent figures for identification, to be permitted resentment. |
| Frustrations: | Arrival of new sibling, physical threats in relation to genital play |
| Personality characteristics and associated behavior: | Differentiation of reality vs. fantasy, curiosity about sex, where babies come from, masturbation; Oedipus situation |
| Mental mechanism and examples: | **Repression:** Forgetting of infantile fears, as of a bogey man. **Reaction Formation:** Behaves in extra brave manner to maintain repression of fears. **Identification:** Of boy with father, girl with mother. |

### Stage Four

| | |
|---|---|
| Age: 6–12 years | Schooler |
| Physical involvement: | Locomotor |
| Psychoanalytical terms: | **Latency, homosexual** |
| Some radius: | Teachers, parents, peers |
| Attitudes and ego strengths: | *Task:* **Industry vs. inferiority, fidelity, skill** |
| Emotional needs: | To develop confidence through social, manual, mental dexterity; to experience success in competition; to experience failure to learn realistic limitations and compensations; and to have adequate adults for identification. |
| Frustrations: | Separation from home |
| Personality characteristics and associated behavior: | Rapid ego development, intellectual development, manual and social dexterity, hero worship, gang phenomenon, disappearance of narcissism: interest in others develops. |

(Continued on next page)

Table 7-3. Continued

| Mental mechanisms and examples: | **Identification:** With schoolteachers, scout leaders, peers of same sex in clique formation. |
|---|---|
| | **Displacement (substitution):** Of attitudes toward parents or to authority figures outside the home. |
| | **Compensation:** For mediocre academic achievement by excelling in sports. |

*Stage Five*

| Age: 12-18 years | Adolescence |
|---|---|
| Physical involvement: | Muscular coordination |
| Psychoanalytical terms: | **Heterosexual** |
| Some radius: | Social cliques, search for mates and partners |
| Attitudes and ego strengths: | *Tasks:* **Identity vs. role diffusion (role confusion)** |
| Emotional needs: | To be allowed emancipatory rebellion against parents: to develop some independence to define sexual identity and role; to develop durable, sustaining relationships outside the family; to be a needed member of a group who makes worthwhile contributions; socially constructive work. |
| Frustrations: | Biological readiness for protection vs. cultural convention |
| Personality characteristics and associated behavior: | Adolescent rebellion, emancipation from parents, adolescent masturbation, homosexual crushes, petting, fantasy, and dating |
| Mental mechanism and examples: | **Identification:** With peers |
| | **Repression:** Of sexual impulses and hostilities |
| | **Sublimation:** Of sexual energy in sports and artistic endeavors |

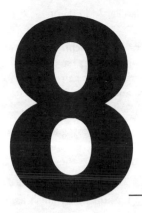

# Disruptive Behavior Disorders

## Attention Deficit Hyperactivity Disorder (ADHD)

In 1926 physician Hans Hoffman wrote in his diary about his school-age son as he was taking care of him for a few days while his wife was in the hospital recovering from giving birth to their second child. Hans noted that his son had cognitive symptoms displayed by his inability to concentrate, his short attention span, and his need to copy repeatedly very easy homework in order to learn it. The boy also demonstrated impulsive behavior. Perhaps these things were happening because his Mom wasn't there; maybe he was a little anxious about sharing his parents with a new sibling. Whatever the cause of his problems, these symptoms applied also to children who had suffered neurologically after the 1917 worldwide flu epidemic and to postencephalitic and brain-damaged children. The disorder was sometimes called "organic driven-ness."

Until the late 1950s, physicians, teachers, and psychiatrists had been seeing this disorder in children and had been treating it as "minimal brain damage"—until they found that there was no definable brain pathology and consequently had to rename it "minimal brain dysfunction," then "hyperkinesis" and "hyperactivity." They noticed that 5% of all children in the United States had this set of symptoms, contrasted to only 1% in England. There, British child psychiatrist and epidemiologist Michael Rutter and his colleagues carefully observed and gathered data that raised serious questions about the validity of the hyperactivity diagnosis, so the disorder was redefined in the late 1970s focusing on the cognitive issues of in-attention and impulsivity rather than on less specific motor manifestations.

ADHD is the most commonly diagnosed childhood disorder, estimated to affect 3–7% of school-age children, and is about four times more common in boys than in girls. However, girls are more typically under-diagnosed because they tend to be more inattentive than hyperactive. A high percentage of children with ADHD have associated learning disabilities, which, with that combination, can cause a major depletion of self-esteem. Whether at home or at school, the child feels he is being criticized for being "too social," for not getting schoolwork completed on time, and for "not listening." This lowered self-esteem often leads to depression. DSM-IV-TR defines ADHD as having some hyperactive, impulsive, or inattentive symptoms causing impairment before age 7 in at least two settings (e.g., school or home), and then there must be clear evidence that there is interference with developmentally appropriate social, academic, or occupational function.

Further defined, it does not occur exclusively during the course of a PDD, schizophrenia or other psychotic disorder, or other mental disorder. Because some studies have shown that physicians have difficulty diagnosing ADHD correctly, at the American Medical Association's annual meeting the Council on Scientific Affairs adopted policies that included continued psychoeducation for physicians.

Toddlers and preschoolers differ from older children by being constantly moving and into everything with more intensity and frequency than the older ones. Impulsivity shows up as impatience, hyperverbalism, and touching everything (including what they're not supposed to touch). Boundaries appear to be undefined for this child.

Until recently, it was believed that the symptoms of ADHD would gradually diminish as the child reached puberty, but several studies have refuted this belief, showing that 20–60% of those adolescents studied still needed treatment. Within this age group there is a high risk for conduct disorder and other antisocial behavior, academic underachievement, low self-esteem, and substance abuse. In the family environment, the ADHD adolescent sometimes has difficulty accepting responsibilities and has disagreements over rights and privileges and permissible social events. Because of low self-esteem, depression is common and can be helped and sometime prevented by the parents' showing a positive attitude. Quite often the parents of an ADHD child/adolescent become frustrated and dysfunctional, which leads to a breakup of the marriage. Parent counseling should definitely be part of the treatment regime.

*Treatment* consists of pharmacotherapy, using stimulants and antidepressants that are targeted to the child's poor attention span, impulsivity or lack of control, and noncompliance with authority directives. Psychostimulant medications, including methylphenidate (Ritalin), dextroamphetamine (Dexedrine), and amphetamine (Adderall), are the most commonly prescribed treatments for ADHD. Catapres may also be used to treat severe impulsiveness. The two most effective treatment modalities for elementary school children with ADHD are a closely monitored medication regime and a combined medication regime with intensive behavioral interventions. Other interventions that are effective are parent counseling and training in child-management skills and classroom behavior modification techniques. The practice guidelines released by the American Academy of Child and Adolescent Psychiatry describe parent education and support as essential to treatment.

An estimated 40% of children diagnosed with ADHD will develop conduct disorder, but the majority of them would be diagnosed with Oppositional Defiant Disorder at an earlier age. Many of the signs and symptoms of ADHD will persist in the adult years in the following ways:

• Having a low stress tolerance leading to a hot temper and impulsivity
• Restlessness, unable to relax easily
• Easily distracted, unable to listen or concentrate
• Unable to complete projects, schoolwork, etc.
• Mood swings (very common in ADHD adults)
• Problems with interpersonal relationships

*Sample of a Behavior Intervention for ADHD Children.* Russell Barkley of the University of Massachusetts Medical Center developed a program for managing defiant and oppositional children who, as he proposed, had an underlying neurophysiological deficiency that caused them to have problems with following rules. His program consisted of 2-hour weekly training sessions provided to individual families and to groups for a 10-week block of time during which they were educated about ADHD and related problems including oppositional-defiant behavior. They learned how to give praise, to ignore inappropriate behavior, and to reward compliance and good behavior with chips or tokens as rewards for compliance on the first command.

*Time-outs* and taking away of tokens earned is another topic that parents learned about. The program stressed that initially a time-out should be used for only two serious forms of defiance that had been problematic for the child. The procedure for the time-out is as follows:

- Issue the command.
- Wait 5 seconds, and then give a warning.
- Wait 5 seconds; take child to time-out area immediately.
- Recommended length of time for time-out is 1-2 minutes per year of age of the child.

Child must meet following before ending time-out:

- Must have served the minimum time assigned.
- Must then remain quiet for a brief period of time—a transition time.
- Must then obey the command given earlier.

Failure to follow the rules of time-out is met with additional punishment such as two spanks on the buttocks or a fine with the tokens previously earned. If the child has many problem behaviors, two of those can be added to the list for reasons for time-out. In a public place it is difficult to manage time-outs, but this program recommends that parents stop before entering the store, office, etc., and review two or three rules that the child has previously defied. Some parents find it helpful to carry a notebook and tell the child that breaking any of these rules will be noted and punishment delayed because of the location.

## Oppositional Defiant and Conduct Disorder

Oppositional Defiant Disorder (ODD) and Conduct Disorder (CD) are termed the adolescent equivalents to the adult antisocial personality disorder. ODD is considered a precursor to conduct disorder as conduct disorder is a precursor to antisocial personality disorder.

### Criteria for ODD Diagnosis

DSM-IV-TR describes ODD as a recurrent problem with defiance, disobedience, and hostility toward authority figures. These problems must last 6 months and include at least four of the following:

- Often loses temper
- Often argues with adults
- Defies authority
- Deliberately annoys individuals
- Blames others for own mistakes
- Is touchy
- Is angry, resentful
- Is spiteful, and vindictive

In addition to six months' duration of symptoms, these behaviors cannot occur exclusively during a mood disorder or psychosis. The behaviors must lead to impairment in school, home, or social functions.

## Conduct Disorder

Teens with conduct disorder lie, steal, cheat, destroy property, and struggle with authority; it is estimated that about 4% of teenagers in a rural setting and 8% in cities have conduct disorders. At this time there is no hard evidence available for the possible etiology. However, a variety of possibilities lead to CD. A genetic vulnerability compounded by an abusive and neglectful upbringing with few models for coping with stress other than through violence and substance abuse, combined with a psychological unwillingness to manage stress in other ways, come together in this disorder.

According to the DSM-IV-TR, in addition to demonstrating a repetitive pattern of behavior that infringes on the rights of others, the child must be doing so in at least three ways over a period of 12 months, and at least one of those ways must have been present in the most recent 6 months. The behaviors are grouped under four major types with a total of fifteen possible specific behaviors. The types are:

• Aggression towards individuals or animals
• Destruction of property
• Deceitfulness or theft
• Serious violation of rules

These behaviors must also lead to an impairment of social, academic, or work functions. Most children meeting the criteria are in late childhood or early adolescence, and few have onset after age 16. The behaviors that result in this diagnosis can be traced back to early childhood, even to 3–6 years old when parents reported aggressiveness, stubbornness, and temper tantrums. When the child enters school, the oppositional behaviors are demonstrated—sometimes by fire setting and stealing. Often the Conduct Disorder diagnosis accompanies other problems such as major depression, schizophrenia, substance abuse, anxiety disorder, ADHD, and PTSD. Girls occasionally have a late onset of CD that usually is associated with promiscuity and substance abuse in the early teens.

## Treatment of ODD and CD

Oppositional Defiant Disorder is not treated with medications unless the child has another psychiatric disorder such as depression, ADHD, or anxiety disorder. Individual therapy with much patience works very well with ODD. Setting safety limits within the therapy session is important, but the therapist needs to stay out of a power struggle with the child.

*Treating Conduct Disorder* is more complex. Usually the referral comes in a time of crisis such as a teenager being arrested. First, the teenager needs a cooling-off period, which can be done at home, in a relative's home, or in a psychiatric hospital. The latter has been a major type of treatment intervention, not necessarily because it's effective, but because it allows for control and a better chance to evaluate the teenager. Medication has been tried in treatment of CD, with neuroleptics and mood stabilizers helping the most in managing acute and chronic irritability and aggression. Individual therapy is usually unacceptable to the problem teenager; teen group therapy may produce better results. In group, the teenager with CD may try bullying others, but he/she needs to be confronted by the therapist, who at the same time needs to be prepared to deal with possibly severe decompensation.

*Traditional family therapy* is not workable with the teenagers, but working with the family system by visiting the home and providing helpful interventions at home is sometimes successful. The prognosis for teens with CD is poor. Only about 25% go on to develop Antisocial Personality Disorder, but the ones with better outcomes grow up to be adults with severe problems, as shown in their poor occupational histories, educational under-achievement, adult sex abuse, psychotic disorders, etc.

## Warning Signs and Symptoms of a Troubled Student

*General Behavior Changes*
• Withdrawn behavior
• Fights with peers or siblings
• Temper outbursts
• Inappropriate giggling/laughter
• Dramatic attention-getting behavior
• Obscene language and gestures
• Increased irritability
• Hyperactivity
• Bizarre and uncontrollable actions
• Extreme apathy
• Erratic behavior
• Hypersensitivity
• Time and place disorientation
• Inappropriate verbal responses
• Depression
• Defensiveness about alcohol/drug use
• Talk about suicide
• Suicide attempt

*School Attendance*
• Classroom tardiness
• First-hour tardiness
• Skipping of classes before and/or after lunch
• All day truancy
• Frequent requests to leave the room

*Academic Performance*
• Drop in grades
• Change in classroom participation
• Inconsistent test grades
• Inconsistent daily work
• Change in penmanship
• Shortened attention span
• Decreased ability to think and solve problems
• Cheating

*Behavior at Home*
- Missing money or objects that could be easily converted into cash
- House supply of liquor or prescription drugs dwindling for no apparent reason
- Increased time spent alone in room
- Possession of bottles of liquor or drug paraphernalia

*Social Problems*
- Deterioration in family relationships and communication
- Running away from home
- Decreased job performance and attendance
- Changing group of friends
- Frequent visits to school counselor or dean's office
- Loss of interest in sports
- Loss of eligibility in sports
- Deterioration of rapport with teachers
- Loss of interest and involvement in hobbies and extracurricular activities

*Legal Problems*
- School suspension
- Possession of alcohol and/or other drugs
- Selling of alcohol and/or other drugs
- Involvement in thefts and/or vandalism
- Arrests for public intoxication, driving while under the influence, or driving while intoxicated

*Physical Warning Signs*
- Frequent visits to school nurse
- Sleeping in class
- Loss of gross motor coordination evidenced by staggering, stumbling
- Vomiting, flushed complexion
- White or pale face
- Puffiness or redness around eyes
- Bloodshot eyes that appear glassy and vague
- Excessive nervousness
- Rapid speech
- Excessive sniffing
- Unusual sores around the nostrils
- Physical injuries
- Slurred speech

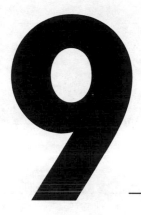

# Child and Adolescent Anxiety Disorders

The American Psychiatric Association defines anxiety as "apprehension, tension, or uneasiness that stems from the anticipation of danger, which may be internal or external." The word anxiety comes from the Latin *anxietas,* "troubled mind." Fear is a psychophysiological response to a real, external, demonstrable threat to safety and life. Anxiety produces the same responses as fear, but the danger is symbolic rather than actual and is associated with unresolved problems and conflicts that are often unconscious.

In 1869, anxiety was referred to as "neurasthenia"; after the Civil War it was described as the "irritable heart syndrome," and after World War I as "effort syndrome." Research over the last 50 years has consistently shown that all children have a large number of fears and anxieties. Two separate studies of several hundred 4–16 year olds reported that each child had an average of 5–8 fears. These fears and anxieties vary not only with age, but also with sex and economic status. Girls report more fears and anxieties than do boys. Anxiety disorders (panic disorder, obsessive-compulsive disorder, generalized anxiety disorders, social phobia, and posttraumatic stress disorder) are, in fact, the most common mental health problems that occur in children and adults. In one large-scale study of 9–17 year olds, as many as 13% had an anxiety disorder in a year. In a 1989 pediatric study (Costello) of 800 patients 7–11 years old, 8.9% met the criteria for at least one anxiety disorder. At least one-third of children with anxiety disorders meet criteria for two or more anxiety disorders.

In anxiety, there is usually a subjective feeling of dread or apprehension ranging from excessive concern about the present or future to feelings of panic. The feeling is accompanied by a variety of physical symptoms such as palpitations, shortness of breath, trembling, skin pallor, and dry mouth. Traditionally, anxiety has been divided into two broad categories according to its etiology: (1) exogenous, when anxieties arise as a result of external events and is psychological, rather than biological, in nature; and (2) endogenous, when it occurs as a result of an underlying biological cause and can have a predictable developmental path, such as in anxiety with panic attacks.

## Separation Anxiety Disorder

This is probably the most common anxiety disorder in young children. A 1992 study of 188 children in an anxiety disorders clinic determined that there was an equal gender distribution and an earlier age of onset (mean of 7.5 years) than in other anxiety disorders, and that these children were more likely to come from low socioeconomic status and single-parent homes. For them the situation is separation from a significant attachment figure. DSM-IV-TR defines Separation Anxiety Disorder as "developmentally inappropriate and excessive anxiety concerning separation from home or from those to whom the individual is attached, as evidenced by three or more of the following:"

- Recurrent excessive distress when separation from home or major attachment figures occur or is anticipated
- Persistent and excessive worry about losing, or about possible harm befalling major attachment figures
- Persistent and excessive worry that an untoward event will lead to separation from a major attachment figure (e.g., getting lost or being kidnapped)
- Persistent reluctance or refusal to go to school or elsewhere because of fear of separation
- Persistent and excessively fearful or reluctant to be alone or without major attachment figures at home or without significant adults in other settings
- Persistent reluctance or refusal to go to sleep without being near a major attachment figure or to sleep away from home
- Repeated nightmares involving the theme of separation
- Repeated complaints of physical symptoms (such as headaches, stomach aches, nausea, or vomiting) when separation from major attachment figure occurs or is anticipated

The duration of the disturbance is at least 4 weeks; the onset is before age 18. The disturbance causes clinically significant distress or impairment in social, academic, occupational, or other important areas of functioning. The disturbance does not occur exclusively during the course of a PDD, schizophrenia, or other psychotic disorder and, in adolescents and adults, is not better accounted for by panic disorder with agoraphobia.

## Treatment

Children with anxiety disorders respond very well to treatment with SSRIs, which are medications that contribute to the relief of the typical physiological symptoms of anxiety and are also quite effective in addressing the cognitive aspects of these disorders, such as worrying, initial insomnia, rumination, decreased concentration, and repetitive or intrusive thinking or behaviors. Antihistamines like Benadryl and Atarax or Vistaril are the two most commonly used medications in treating anxiety disorders in children.

## Instruments for Assessment of Anxiety in Children and Adolescents

There are diverse measures available to assess symptoms in children. One is the Schedule for Affective Disorders and Schizophrenia for School-Age Children (K-SADS). This is a semi-structured interview of both parents and child to identify the presence and severity of a broad range of symptoms. Based on the interview results, DSM-IV diagnoses can be made for affective and other disorders. Other diagnostic interviews available include the

Diagnostic Interview for Children and Adolescents-Revised (Weiner et al., 1987), the NMH Diagnostic Interview for Children (Chambers et al., 1985), the Anxiety Disorders Interview Schedule for Children (Silverman & Nelles, 1988), and the Anxiety Rating for Children-Revised (Bernstein et al., 1996). There are more assessment tools, depending on the circumstance.

## Obsessive-Compulsive Disorder (OCD)

Unwanted, intrusive, and repetitive thoughts (obsessions) and rituals (compulsions) occurring out of a feeling of urgent need characterize this disorder. At least one-third to one-half of adult cases start between the ages of 10–12 years old. This is the fourth most common neurobiological illness, with 1 in 40 adults and 1 in 200 children having a lifetime occurrence. Common obsessions are: concern with order, counting, fear of acting on aggressive impulses (30%), dirt, germs, and contamination (35%). Typical compulsions we see most often include: repetitive handwashing (75%), checking and rechecking, repetitive actions such as stepping only on the cracks in the sidewalk, and concern with arranging. This neurological illness is believed to affect specific pathways in the brain using the serotonin transmitter. There is a relationship between a subgroup of children with OCD and tic disorders.

## Panic Disorder

This is characterized by feelings of extreme fear and dread that strike unexpectedly and repeatedly for no apparent reason, often accompanied by intense physical symptoms such as dizziness, abdominal distress, chest pain, pounding heart, and shortness of breath. This is differentiated from a generalized anxiety attack because there's no apparent reason, and no identifiable worry that brought it on. Panic disorder can also include agoraphobia, so this needs to be assessed when making the diagnosis. Four or more of the following symptoms may develop abruptly and peak in 10 minutes:

- Palpitations, pounding heart, or accelerated heart rate
- Sweating
- Trembling or shaking
- Sensations of shortness of breath or smothering
- Feeling of choking
- Chest pain or discomfort
- Nausea or abdominal distress
- Feeling of dizziness, unsteadiness; lightheaded or faint
- Feelings of unreality or being detached from self
- Fear of going crazy or losing control
- Fear of dying
- Numbness (paresthesia)
- Chills or hot flushes

## Panic Disorder with Agoraphobia

This refers to anxiety about being in places or situations from which escape might be difficult or embarrassing. Certain situations are avoided or are endured with marked distress or with anxiety about having a panic attack or require a companion to be near. Other mental disorders such as social phobia, OCD, PTSD, and separation anxiety need to be ruled out. Treatment consists of behavior modification and individual and family therapy.

## Phobias

*Social phobias* are characterized by extreme fear of being embarrassed or scrutinized. Exposure to the situation almost invariably provokes immediate anxiety response. Children do not always recognize that this fear is unreasonable.

*Specific phobias* refer to an excessive fear of an object or situation, such as heights, animals, places, noises, etc. In individuals under 18, the symptoms must have been present for at least 6 months. The five types of specific phobias are:

- Animal Type
- Natural Environmental Type
- Blood-Injection-Injury Type
- Situational Type (e.g., airplanes, elevators, enclosed places)
- Other Type (e.g., phobic avoidance of situations that may lead to choking, vomiting, or contracting an illness; in children, avoidance of loud sounds or costumed characters.)

## Posttraumatic Stress Disorder (PTSD)

All children experience a crisis of some degree every day in their young lives. To a child, it is a crisis when they can't find their homework, they can't find a matching sock, their best friend didn't play with them yesterday, etc. When children are unable to cope with the crisis and it begins to dictate how they sleep, eat, think, feel, and behave, then the crisis has caused and continues to produce trauma which interrupts their normal growth and development. In younger children, scary dreams of traumatizing events can turn into nightmares that are played out throughout the day because they don't realize they're reliving the event. They may feel that their lives will be so short they'll never make it to adulthood and may even believe that they have an ability to foresee future untoward events.

PTSD can occur at any age and usually occurs within 3 months after a trauma. The duration of the symptoms varies, but in half the cases, complete recovery occurs within 3 months after the symptoms begin. In children, the response to the traumatizing event must involve disorganized or agitated behavior to meet the criteria for the DSM-IV-TR diagnosis of PTSD, which links anxiety to a catastrophic event such as rape, assault, combat, earthquake, airplane crash, act of terrorism, or war. The anxiety associated with the event brings about general arousal, such as hypervigilance, and diminishes the range of emotions and interest in significant activities.

The kinds of experiences or conditions that can seriously traumatize children are: 1) victimization, which includes assault, robbery, rape, serious accidents, and incest; 2) loss such as divorce, moving, changing schools, leaving home, and separation from family member(s); and 3) family pathology, which includes incest, chemical dependency, abuse, domestic violence, and other forms of dysfunction.

The team of Coleman, Butcher, and Carson (1980) have identified four categories of family dysfunction that are associated with higher incidences of psychological disorders, leading to physical illness and various maladaptive behaviors. These four categories are:

- *Inadequate families* that lack the physical or psychological resources for coping with normal stressors.

- *Anti-social families* that have different values from those of their communities, which may encourage undesirable behaviors.

- *Discordant and disturbed families* with fraudulent interpersonal contracts and disturbances, e.g., fighting, gross irrationality, or enmeshment of the family in parental conflicts.

- *Disrupted families* that have inadequately adjusted to the loss of family members through death, divorce, and/or separation.

## Assessment

Relatives, teachers, childcare workers, parents, friends—all can help put together the information for making the assessment.

Nonverbal signs of PTSD in children who are younger include:

- Sleep disturbances continuing more than several days, wherein actual dreams of the trauma may or may not appear;

- Clinging behavior or anxiety from separating, such as reluctance to go back to school;

- Phobias about distressing stimuli such as individuals, places, and events that remind the child of the precipitating event;

- Conduct disturbances at home or school that are responses to anxiety and frustration;

- Doubts about the self, including comments about body confusion, self-worth, and desire to withdraw.

## Treatment

The best course of action is to provide a safe place for the child to discharge feelings, reactions, and negative behaviors so as to restore him/her to previous levels of functioning.

*Table 9-1. Five key points for treatment of PTSD*

- Assess the child as soon as possible after the critical incident.
- Build a rapport with the child.
- Involve family as much as possible.
- Explore and correct inaccurate attributions regarding the trauma.
- Use play therapy, art therapy, music therapy, cognitive behavior therapy, group therapy, sand tray, family therapy, and any combination thereof which seems appropriate to assist the child to recovery.

## Pharmacotherapy (See also chapter 12)

This usually consists of benzodiazepines and antidepressants, but the choice needs to be carefully made depending on the particular condition and the side effects of the chosen medication. The use of either benzodiazepines and antidepressants in the management of anxiety disorders in children remains poorly studied and understood.

# Overanxious Disorder of Childhood (Generalized Anxiety Disorder)

Even though more than half of the adults presenting for treatment for generalized anxiety disorder report onset of symptoms in their childhood or adolescence, onset after age 20 is common. In children and adolescents, the anxieties and worries often concern the quality of their performance or competence at school or in sporting events. They may have excessive concerns about punctuality or catastrophic events. The child may be overly conforming and a perfectionist as well as over zealous in seeking approval and reassurance. One of the following symptoms (as opposed to 3 or more for adults) must be present for more days than not over the past 6 months:

- Restlessness
- Easily fatigued
- Difficulty in concentrating or remembering
- Irritability
- Muscle tension
- Sleep disturbance

## Assessment

There are diverse measures available to assess symptoms in children. One is the Schedule for Affective Disorders and Schizophrenia for School-Age Children (K-SADS). This is a semi-structured interview of both parents and child to identify the presence and severity of a broad range of symptoms. Based on the interview results, DSM-IV diagnoses can be made for affective and other disorders.

There are many diagnostic interviews available, including the Diagnostic Interview for Children and Adolescents-Revised (Welner et al., 1987); the Anxiety Disorders Interview (Silverman & Nelles, 1988); the Multidimensional Anxiety Scale for Children (1996), and the current popular one, the Manifest Anxiety Scale.

# Bereavement (see also Chapter 11)

Kubler-Ross outline five major stages of bereaving: denial, anger, bargaining, depression, and acceptance, which apply to losses as well. In addition, Frears and Schneider (1981) present the following six-stage model:

- Initial awareness (including shock, loss of equilibrium, and lowered resistance to infection)
- Strategies to overcome loss (including adaptive defense cycles of holding on and letting go)

- Awareness of loss (including exploration of extent of loss and its ramifications, such as loneliness, helplessness, and exhaustion
- Completions (healing, acceptance, resolution, and freeing the energy invested in the loss)
- Empowering the self (in areas that were out of balance prior to the loss)
- Transcending the loss (growth following completions and re-balancing)

Children under ten have not developed their ability to recognize, understand, and resolve loss. The following chart illustrates Wass's correlation of death concepts relating to development (1984).

*Table 9-2. Development of Concept of Death*

| Life Period | Predominant Death Concepts |
| --- | --- |
| **Infancy** | No concept of death |
| **Late infancy, Early childhood** | Death is reversible; a temporary restriction, departure, or sleep |
| **Middle childhood Late or preadolescence** | Death is irreversible; external-internal, physiological explanations |
| **Preadolescent Adolescent, adult** | Death is irreversible, universal, personal but distant, natural; physiological and has theological explanations |

What we can do as therapists is provide a safe place for the child to discharge feelings, reactions, and negative behaviors so as to restore him/her to previous levels of functioning.

# 10 Other Psychiatric Disorders in Children

This chapter will include disorders from several categories of the DSMIV that haven't been discussed previously in this manual.

## Stereotypic Movement Disorder

This disorder consists of repetitive motor behavior that interferes with normal activities or results in bodily injury (self-inflicted) that requires medical treatment. This disorder is not accounted for by tics, hair-pulling compulsion, substance abuse, or a medical condition, and commonly occurs in association with mental retardation. In fact, there is a prevalence of 2.3% of self-injurious behavior in the mentally retarded as a population and a 25% prevalence in mentally retarded adults who are institutionalized. The onset of self-injurious behavior may follow a stressful event or painful medical condition such as an ear infection, which might lead to head banging Head banging is 3 times more likely in males than in females, who are more likely to self-bite.

A few approaches have been successful in decreasing the occurrence of stereotypes. One type is manipulating the setting or antecedent events, such as the environment, the activity or objects present, whether or not the individual is alone or socially interacting, and the use of exercise. Several studies, though, have indicated that manipulation of the antecedent events exclusive of drug use was only minimally effective. Another method has been using aversive techniques including electric shock, physical restraint, physical consequences such as a slap, aversive music, water mist sprayed in the face, and over correction, which is a technique requiring the practice of alternate forms of responding. The latter has been generally effective in reducing stereotypes.

Another method is the use of positive procedures involving differential reinforcement of other (DRO) and differential reinforcement of incompatible (DRI) behaviors. However, this method works best in combination with the use of some of the other techniques mentioned. Another recommended technique is manipulation of sensory stimulation, which also works in combination with other methods.

## Selective Mutism

This disorder occurs in less than 1% of children and usually before the age of 5. Children with this disorder may communicate by gestures, altered voice, or short monotone utterances. The disorder usually lasts for only a few months. Associated features are excessive shyness, clinging, negativism. DSM-IV criteria for this diagnosis includes:

- Persistent failure to speak in specific social situations (e.g., at school or with playmate where speaking is expected, despite speaking in other situations).
- Disturbance interferes with educational or occupational achievement or with social communication.
- Must last for at least 1 month and isn't limited to the first month of school when the child will be meeting new friends.

Do NOT diagnosis this if the failure to speak is due to a lack of knowledge of or comfort with the spoken language required in the social situation, if the disturbance is better accounted for by embarrassment relating to having a communications disorder such as stuttering, or if it occurs during a psychotic disorder, schizophrenia, or a PDD.

## Reactive Attachment Disorder

This disorder begins before the age of 5 and is very uncommon. Marked disturbance and developmentally inappropriate social relatedness is present and is associated with grossly pathological care. Two types of this disturbance are:

- *Inhibited type:* the persistent failure to initiate and to respond to most social interactions in a developmentally appropriate way.
- *Disinhibited type:* indiscriminate sociability or a lack of selectivity in the choice of attachment figures.

In the first type mentioned, the child shows a pattern of hypervigilance, excessive inhibitions, or highly ambivalent responses (e.g., frozen watchfulness, resistance to comfort, or a mixture of approach and avoidance). In the second type, the pattern shows very diffuse attachments as mentioned above. By definition, the condition is associated with: grossly pathological care that may show persistent disregard for the child's emotional needs for comfort, stimulation, and affection; or persistent disregard for the child's basic physical needs; or repeated changes of the primary caregiver, preventing formation of stable attachments. Improvement or remission may take place providing that an appropriately supportive environment is provided. Otherwise, no change in the disordered child is to be expected.

## Mental Disorders and Their Impact

Serious mental disorders in children are characterized by the duration, intensity, and interference effect of their symptom behaviors, that is, its impact on other significant areas of the child's life. For example, a child who cannot write his schoolwork or join in games with peers because he is so involved in nail biting clearly needs a mental health assessment. Among these are:

### Adjustment Disorders

An estimated 5–10% of all children struggle with adjustment disorders; among children under 12, the disorders are seen more frequently in preschoolers and in young school-aged children, whose coping abilities are not fully developed. Adjustment disorders are defined as transient disturbances of normal functioning due to identifiable stressors, with symptoms that are usually temporary but intense, such as insomnia, bedwetting, regressive behavior, refusal to eat, overeating, etc. Often the symptoms appear after a stressful event that may be clearly significant to the child and NOT to the adult.

### Pervasive Development Disorders (PDD)

Symptoms are bizarre and extreme. Sometimes children with symptoms are mislabeled as retarded. Symptoms consist of poor interpersonal relationships, confused personal identity, poorly developed speech or use of language, inconsistent performance in school, hyperactivity, marked resistance to change in environment, and self-mutilating or self-stimulating behaviors (see chapter 3).

## Psychophysiological Disorders

*Asthma* affects 2% of children; *GI disorders,* about 10%. Symptoms can vary from mild discomforts to life-threatening disorders such as ulcerative colitis. The child's internalized anxiety causes physical discomfort and may lead to physiologic damage. This child is usually referred to the school nurse for headaches, stomachache, diarrhea, and difficulty in breathing. Frequent crises or uncontrolled periods among children who have epilepsy or diabetes are included in this category of disorders.

*Enuresis* is usually defined as the involuntary or voluntary passage of urine in children over 5 years of age—2 times a week the child either bed wets or wets his clothing for 3 consecutive months—or the enuresis results in clinically significant distress or impairment in social, academic, or other important areas of functioning. The diagnosis is not made until child is at least 5 years old.

- Primary — always existed without periods of dryness beginning at age 5
- Secondary — consistently dry for a period of 6–12 months before beginning to wet at age 5 or anytime after
- Subtypes:
  - Nocturnal — wetting occurs at night during sleep (bed-wetting)
  - Diurnal — wetting occurs during the day
  - Nocturnal and diurnal — combination
  - Mode of inheritance remains unknown
  - Children with enuresis have a reduced functional bladder capacity; as a result they void more frequently during the day (not anatomically reduced)

Treatment/management is usually behavioral modification combined with tricyclic antidepressants (particularly Tofranil), which can be effective on a short-term basis but the child may develop a tolerance after 6 weeks.

**NOTE:** A child is not diagnosed with enuresis if he/she: (1) has a neurogenic bladder, (2) has a general medical condition causing polyuria or urgencies (i.e., diabetes), or (3) has a urinary tract infection.

*Encopresis* is defined as repeated voluntary or involuntary passage of feces into inappropriate places not acceptable in that individual's sociocultural setting. It must occur at least one time per month for 3 consecutive months, and the chronological age must be at least 4 years old or developmentally equivalent. The behavior cannot be due exclusively to the direct physiological effects of substance (i.e., a laxative) or a general medical condition, except through a mechanism involving constipation. The prevalence of encopresis is estimated to be 1% of 5-year-olds and more common in males.

### Types of encopresis (according to DSM-IV)
- With constipation and overflow incontinence
- Without constipation and overflow incontinence
  - Associated features
    - Symptom of childhood stress
    - Adjustment difficulties
    - Lowered self-esteem
    - Social ostracism by peers
    - Anger, punishment, rejection by caregivers
    - Deliberate or accidental smearing of feces
    - Sometimes related to conduct disorders or oppositional defiance disorder
    - School/family transitions

  - Diagnostic Tests: Rule out diarrheal disorders, Hirshsprung disease, hypothyroidism, chronic codeine or phenothiazine use, disease/obstruction of the intestines; then a rectal biopsy, UA, and urine culture.

  - Treatment/management consists of complete bowel clean out, light mineral oil for several months, and daily routine of sitting on the toilet for 10 minutes to develop bowel pattern, giving lots of praise.

*Tourette's disorder (or Tourette's syndrome)* is sometimes referred to as TS and is a complex inherited neurological disorder characterized by motor and phonic tics as well as by obsessions and compulsions. These tics may appear simultaneously or at different periods during the illness, many times a day, recurrently throughout a period of more than a year. During that 1-year period, there is never a tic-free period of more than 3 consecutive months. There is significant impairment in social, occupational, and other areas of functioning. More than 100,000 people in the United States have TS. The onset typically happens between the ages of 5–10, peaking in severity by age 10, and the tics aren't due to the direct effects of a substance (e.g., stimulants) or a general medical condition such as Huntington disease or post-viral encephalitis.

According to the DSM-IV-TR, the anatomical location, number, frequency, complexity, and severity of the tics change over time and typically involve the head and other parts of the body, such as the torso and limbs. The vocal tics include various words or sounds such as clicks, grunts, yelps, barks, sniffs, snorts, and coughs. Corprolalia, a complex vocal tic involving the use of obscenities, is present in less than 10% of the cases but is not rare.

- Complications of TS include physical injury such as blindness due to retinal detachment (from head banging or striking oneself), orthopedic problems (from knee bending, neck jerking, or head turning), and skin problems from picking. TS occurs in approximately 4–5/10,000 and is 1.5–3 times more common in males. The median age of onset is 7 years and the disorder usually lasts for a lifetime with remissions. About 50–90% of TS patients will have symptoms of ADHD, and up to 50% of them will have OCD or some traits of it.

- TS cannot be diagnosed by lab work or blood work, and sometimes it's many years before a diagnosis can be made after the symptoms appear. Other problems such as eyestrain, stress, and seasonal allergies can interfere with making a diagnosis. Treatment of TS consists of neuroleptic medications such as Haldol, Prolixin, and Orap. Since these drugs tend to have negative side effects such as muscle rigidity, sedation, tardive dyskinesia, etc., a newer group of neuroleptics are now being used that have fewer side effects. Those drugs are: Risperdal, Navane, and Zyprexa. Clonidine, an antihypertensive, is also being used to avert motor tics. In addition, antidepressants (Anafranil and Prozac), tricyclic antidepressants (Norpramin, Tofranil) and psychostimulants (Ritalin and dexedrine) are used, depending on the symptoms presenting. The latter two categories are useful in alleviating ADHD symptoms, decreasing anxieties, and improving attention deficits.

The clinical specialist role with an individual diagnosed with TS is to provide support, comfort, assistance with physical care, building self-esteem, and educating the patient, teachers, family, and staff. Monitoring medication side effects and continually assessing behavior will all be very important. You may have to help the staff to develop interventions for behavior problems as well.

*Trichotillomania* is an impulse-control disorder that has the diagnostic criteria of a recurrent pulling out of one's hair resulting in noticeable hair loss. Common sites of hair may include any part of the body, but the most common sites are the scalp, eyebrows, and eyelashes. Pleasure is derived from the hair pulling, and it usually occurs after an increasing sense of tension. Trichophagia (eating hair) may accompany the disorder. The age of onset is usually before young adulthood but peaks around ages 5–8 years and age 13 and appears to be more common in females. Some individuals have urges to pull hair from others and from carpets, sweaters, etc. Individuals with this disorder may also have mood disorders, anxiety disorders, or mental retardation.

## Childhood Schizophrenia

Before 1980, autism and schizophrenia were both listed under the term childhood schizophrenia. DSM-III changed that and classified them as two separate disorders with one important difference: that on clinical examination of autistic children, no auditory or visual hallucinations or delusions are present, whereas most schizophrenic children do have those symptoms. Childhood-onset schizophrenia is diagnosed using the same criteria used to diagnose adults, with symptoms including thought disorder, hallucinations, delusions, socially impaired relationships, and a presence of unusual affects The incidence of schizophrenia in the general population is 1% but rises considerably with parental diagnosis of schizophrenia.

In 1967, Rutter made a distinction between autism (very early onset) and childhood-onset schizophrenia (average age of onset at 8 or 9 years). The latter is extremely rare and has increasing prevalence with age. However, Anna Freud, Bleuler, and Winnecott all stress the importance of the early phase of the child's life when he/she needs a satisfactory breastfeeding experience as well as ego support from the mother's identification and bonding with the baby in the first 2 years of life. This leads to development of good mental health and competence. When Sigmund Freud speaks of the confidence and success of the mother's favorite, he is talking in "self" rather than "ego" terms and stressing that it is the self that develops the sense of invulnerability.

In 1968, an Icelander named Karlsson described a group of "genetic carriers" with thought disorder who were descendants of many generations of schizophrenic "stock" but who currently showed high ability and achievement in art, science, and politics. He wondered if these creative individuals could be regarded as "non-penetrant schizophrenics." In 1963 another researcher, Barron, had said that the answer was not genetic but was instead the degree of ego resilience and integration. According to the DSM-IV-TR, the first-degree biological relatives of individuals with schizophrenia have a risk for schizophrenia that is 10 times greater than that of the general population.

The onset of schizophrenia typically occurs between the late teens and the mid-thirties with rare cases in adolescence. There have been reported cases in children with age of onset at 5 or 6 years. Before age 3, if symptoms have begun, the child is diagnosed as having an autistic disorder. Schizophrenia can also begin later in life (e.g., after age 45). To make a diagnosis of schizophrenia in children is very difficult, because the delusions and hallucinations may be less elaborated as in adults and visual hallucinations may be more common. There are many disorders where disorganized speech is observed (e.g., communication disorders, PDD) and when there is disorganized behavior.

Whereas schizophrenia was previously commonly diagnosed in children, now obsessive-compulsive disorder (OCD), pervasive development disorder (PDD), affective disorders, posttraumatic stress disorders (PTSD), and atypical psychosis are all more common. Hallucinations in children may occur in a number of nonpsychotic conditions and are less likely in adolescents. Differential diagnoses will include conduct disorders with later social withdrawals, mood disorders with both manic and psychotic depressive episodes, pervasive developmental disorders (with severe language disorders), obsessive-compulsive disorders, and organically based disorders such as substance induced, tumors, infection, and autoimmune disorders.

*Schizophrenia's disturbance* exists for about 6 months and has at least 1 month of active-phase symptoms (i.e., two or more) of the following: delusions, hallucinations, disorganized speech, grossly disorganized or catatonic behavior, negative symptoms such as affective flattening, alogia, or avolition.

NOTE: Alogia (poverty of speech) is manifested by brief and empty replies. Avolition is characterized by an inability to initiate and persist in goal-directed activities. There are five subtypes of schizophrenia: paranoid, disorganized, catatonic, undifferentiated, and residual.

*The positive symptoms of schizophrenia* reflect an excess of distortion of normal functions, and the negative symptoms reflect a loss of normal function (as in the affective flattening mentioned previously). Childhood-onset schizophrenia must be distinguished from childhood presentations combining disorganized speech (from a communication disorder) and disorganized behavior (from ADHD). The child must also have failed to achieve the expected level of interpersonal, academic, or occupational achievement. If there's a history of PDD or autistic disorder, the additional diagnosis of schizophrenia is made only if prominent delusions or hallucinations have been present for at least a month.

*Other psychotic disorders to rule out* when diagnosing schizophrenia are: (1) schizophreniform disorder, (2) schizoaffective disorder, (3) delusional disorder, (4) brief psychotic disorder, (5) shared psychotic disorder, (6) psychotic disorder due to a general medical condition, (7) substance-induced psychotic disorder, and (8) psychotic disorder NOS.

There are diverse measures available to assess symptoms in children. One is the Schedule for Affective Disorders and Schizophrenia for School-Age Children (K-SADS). This is a semi-structured interview of both parents and 6–17-year-old child to identify the presence and severity of a broad range of symptoms. Based on the interview results, DSM-IV diagnoses can be made for affective and other disorders. The Behavioral Screening Questionnaire is for identifying preschool age children with emotional disorders, and the Child Screening Inventory is aimed at finding emotional disorders in children 6–18 years. The Functional Interview Schedule for Children assesses events as they relate to the behavior, and the Interview Schedule for Children emphasizes symptoms related to depression.

*Treatment for schizophrenia* consists of the older antipsychotics such as Thorazine, Haldol, Mellaril, Prolixin, and Navane, which have been shown to be affective but have short-term side effects such as extrapyramidal symptoms (EPS) and tardive dyskinesia. Newer atypical antipsychotics are becoming popular because they have fewer side effects. Some of them are: Risperidone, Olanzeprine, Quentepine, and Clozabine.

# Delusional Disorders

Delusional disorders are common features of both organic and nonorganic psychotic disorders. They consist of false, fixed beliefs or perceptions not based on reality or that are misinterpretations and distortions of reality:

*Nursing Interventions include:*
• Establishing trust.
• Assurance of safety.
• Assessing source, stressors, and meanings of delusions.
• Reasoning or argument is often useless.
• Acknowledge the process of the client's experience rather than the content of the delusions, i.e., "It must be frightening to think people are trying to harm you."
• Acknowledge the plausible elements of the delusion.
• Decrease paranoia by remaining open and honest while respecting the client's experience.
• Remember that delusions often have some basis in fact, occasionally more than we think. Don't forget the saying, "Just because you're paranoid doesn't mean they aren't out to get you."
• Become familiar with the entire DSM as well as current nursing interventions. This mastery is an important part of the practice of a CNS.

# Childhood Depression

Childhood is thought of as a happy time in life, free from worry, but children can and do suffer from depression, an illness once thought of as affecting adults only. Sometimes, painful events can lead to depression in children; other times, it seems to occur without reason. Like adults, children can have moody times, but if a depressed mood lingers, it can become an illness and lead to serious consequences. According to the American Psychiatric Association, 1 in 10 children ages 6 to 12 suffers from a depressive illness and is unable to escape persistent feelings of sadness. It is estimated that three to six million children may suffer from depression at some point and may be at increased risk for suicide.

A depressed child may run away, set fires, abuse drugs, withdraw from others, become lethargic, and lose self-esteem. The two choices children have when they face depression are withdrawing further or acting out. They may become frustrated, feel hopeless and sad; these feelings can turn into anger or hostility that can lead to aggressive or troublesome behaviors. A child may not be able to tell how he feels and instead lets you know through his/her behavior. Two of the most common types of depression are depressive episodes and major depressive disorder. Depressive episodes usually milder, transient, and related to a specific stress or loss; they may last only a few days or weeks. Major depressive disorder may begin at any age and often follows a severe psychosocial stressor. Up to 15% of individuals with major depressive disorder die by suicide.

## Signs of Childhood Depression

- Aggression, temper tantrums, antisocial behavior, uncooperative
- Increased irritability
- Poor concentration, low energy, fatigue, persistent boredom
- Low self-esteem
- Unstable moods
- Use of illegal substances
- Increased truancy and poor academic performance
- Noticeable changes in sleeping and eating patterns
- Persistent sadness
- Increased physical complaints
- Recurring thoughts of death or suicide

The signs of teenage depression are similar to the signs seen in younger children but appear to be more intense. The feeling that life is a big disappointment and not worth living is more common in teenagers who are struggling with relationships, life plans, career choices, physiological changes, and self-esteem.

Teenage depression is extremely painful and debilitating and is often accompanied by thoughts of suicide. It is more prevalent among girls than boys. In the United States, suicide is one of the leading causes of death among adolescents, and The Centers for Disease Control and Prevention reported that children age 10–14 are committing suicide twice as often as 20 years ago. Suicide by using guns has increased. If symptoms last for more than a few weeks or if the child becomes dangerous to self or others, the child should get a complete diagnostic evaluation from an physician to rule out any physical problems. If no physical problems are present, the child should be psychologically evaluated by a psychiatrist, psychologist, or other licensed professional familiar with children.

In preschool children, depression is rare but does occur. This is a time when children are having to separate from parents and be comfortable in a school environment with new friends. If the child's home situation is stressful due to family addiction, physical or sexual abuse at home, a high degree of family discord, recent death in the family, recent birth of a sibling, parental separation/divorce, recent moving away from friends or into a new community, the symptoms of depression will begin to emerge. Early/middle school children are more likely to show depression after age 10. They may have physical complaints, complaints of feeling "down in the dumps," and may become irritable and isolative.

## Treatment of Childhood Depression

There is sparse history of treatment of children with depression, so information has been gained from research of treatment of adult depression. It has been shown, though, that depressive symptoms and associated features continue from childhood through adolescence and into adulthood. Treatment may consist of outpatient counseling, inpatient hospitalization, medications, family therapy, group therapy, and any combination of treatments mentioned here. There is also concern over the possible permanent effects that drugs may have on growth, intelligence, development, and nonsymptomatic behaviors. In addition, possible side effects that are temporary, such as physiological changes or minor discomforts—and more severe effects such as seizures or death—are to be considered. Withdrawal from medications can produce side effects as well. Some of the following treatments being used are listed below:

*Response contingent reinforcement* increases the level of pleasant activities in which depressed individuals engage, thus decreasing the depressive symptoms. Treatment includes asking the patients to self-monitor their moods and activities and to identify the positive reinforcing activities which are associated with their positive affect.

*Social skills training* is sometimes used to increase the person's ability to obtain reinforcement from others. The patient is treated individually and provided with instructions, modeling by the therapist, role-playing, feedback, and planned activities where the patient has to initiate conversation, respond to others, refuse requests of others, make requests, etc.

*Interpersonal psychotherapy* focuses on interpersonal relationships, social adjustments, and mastery of social roles through nonjudgmental exploration of feelings, reflective listening, development of insight, direct advice, and elicitation and active questioning by the therapist. This type of therapy is based on the general observation that the social role performance of depressed patients is dysfunctional. However, this focus on roles is not as useful in working with depressed children.

*Combined psychotherapy* with medication has been shown to be more effective than either treatment alone. Psychotherapy tends to alter problems of living and social dysfunction, whereas medication alters the regressive signs. The combined treatment provides broader coverage in the range of symptoms that are improved, but there are different schools of thought about this, particularly in the treatment of children.

*Medications:* Although the newest class of SSRIs (selective serotonin reuptake inhibitors) such as Prozac, Paxil, Zoloft, Luvox, and Celexa are very effective in adults, the FDA has not approved them for use with children. Studies are showing, however, that there are fewer side effects from them than from TCAs (tricyclic antidepressants). In addition, adrenergic agents such as Wellbutrin, Remeron, and Effexor are being used because of their safer side effects. Most research on the treatment of childhood depression is on medications; however, the guidelines are not clear and greater caution is needed in the administration of medications. It has been found that medication has unclear effects in treating depressed adolescents.

*Cognitive behavior models* have been the ones most used of the treatment techniques for depressed children. In these models, the subjects received training in self-control skills, relaxation, self-evaluation and self-reinforcement, examination of their cognitive distortions and faulty beliefs, and problem solving. Research has shown that Beck's Cognitive Therapy applies to children and that depressed children show the negative bias in their view of the world, themselves, and the future. At the core of this theory is the negative "cognitive triad," which refers to those characteristics that lead to depressive symptoms. The cognitive therapy approach is designed to alter negatively based cognitions by training depressed patients to recognize the connections between their thoughts, affect, and behavior; to monitor their negative thoughts; to challenge their thoughts with evidence; and to substitute more reality-based interpretations for their usual cognitions. They are also assigned to engage in specific behaviors outside of treatment.

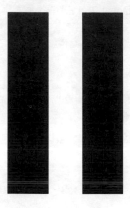

# Other Issues

## Suicide of Youth

Youth suicide is a major concern in the US. On any given day, approximately 1,000 adolescents will attempt suicide. Of those, 18 will be successful. On that same day, 36 young adults between 20 and 24 years of age will also succeed. Teenagers at increased risk of suicide are any who have had a parent or friend who has committed suicide, any teen who abused drugs or alcohol, and any teen who is self-critical and an overachiever.

Among young suicide victims, two-thirds have had counseling and one-third have been hospitalized. One-third of all runaways are acutely suicidal. Fifty percent of all youth suicide victims are from "broken" homes; however, intact families also experience suicide of a child, sometimes because life is very hectic in the busy family and quality communication time averages about 10 minutes per day for each child with the parent. Also, if a parent commits suicide, the possibility of suicide by the child is increased by 900%.

Preadolescent suicide is less common and can probably be explained by the following reasons:

- Children under ten have a very undeveloped concept of death, often seeing it as reversible and not as something they do to themselves.
- They seldom have the ready means or equipment to carry out the act.
- The process of introjection and identification with a lost love object, often seen as one of the dynamics of suicide among the young, only becomes dominant in adolescence.
- The "phenomenology of depression" changes at puberty so that feelings of helplessness, hopelessness, and lonliness are only then converted into a suicidal intent. The child is more likely to express depression by acting out or running away.

Our Western culture is primed to believe that children don't kill themselves and will exhaust every alternative explanation before society concedes that a suicide has happened. Some researchers believe that the real suicide rate for very young children is probably much higher than the reported figures. The child will seldom leave a note or other communication with intent. Sometimes, without ready means for self-destruction, the suicide will be thought to be an accident—perhaps jumping or "accidentally" getting into parent's medications or household chemicals.

Symptoms of increased suicidal risk:

- Hints of "I'd be better off dead," "Nothing matters; it's no use," "No one will miss me anyway."
- When the person has trouble concentrating.
- Increased appetite and weight gain or decreased appetite and weight loss.
- Withdrawal from friends and family.
- Sudden efforts to "make peace."
- Sudden mood changes or behavior change; restlessness.
- Increased need for naps and/or sleeping later.
- Poor sleep with early wake up.
- Loss of interest in pleasurable activities.
- Acting-out behaviors.
- Recent accident or close call.
- Sudden "cleaning house," giving away possessions.
- Depression for more than two weeks.

*Substance abuse:* According to the Fifth Special Report to the U.S. Congress on Alcohol and Health (1983), as many as 80% of people who attempt suicide have been drinking at the time.

According to the American Psychiatric Association pamphlet "Teen Suicide," the ratio of suicide success rate for male to female is 4–1. However, young women <u>attempt</u> suicide 6–8 times more frequently.

## Interventions for the Suicidal Child or Adolescent

- Assessment
  - History
  - Family problems
  - School performance
  - Peer group issues
  - Personality and behavior
  - Interview behavior
  - Play therapy

- Determination of Lethality
  - How serious is intent?
  - Does child have a method?
  - Probability of rescue?
  - Does anyone know?
  - When?
  - What might change his mind?

- Consider Legal, Ethical, and Clinical Responsibilities
  - Know your limitations and boundaries of competence.
  - Be well versed in crisis intervention, suicide prevention skills and theory knowledge.

- Understand procedures for voluntary and involuntary hospitalizations.
- Know legal ramifications applying to minors.
- Be clear with client and straightforward in times of crisis.
- Be cognizant of suicide issues through all classes of professional relationship.
- In clinics and agency settings, make sure lines of responsibility are clearly delineated.
- If client possesses weapons or other items that enhance lethality, make sure items are made unavailable.
- Acknowledge client's despair and try to communicate realistic hopes.
- Communicate caring and willingness to listen to his/her pain.
- Encourage client to share in the responsibility for decisions and actions
- Cultivate a support network with and for the client to build a wider resource of caring people

- Document all steps you take in crisis cases
  - Play therapy
  - Individual/group therapy
  - Medication/psychiatrist/APN
  - Family counseling
  - Psychological testing
  - School, parents, therapist, hospital; consultation
  - Suicide contract, crisis phone number given to child

# Child Abuse

California Penal Code 11165.6 describes child abuse as:

> a physical injury which is inflicted by other than accidental means on a child by another person. "Child Abuse" also means the sexual abuse of a child or any act of omission proscribed by Section 273a (willful cruelty or unjustifiable punishment of a child) or 273d (unlawful corporal punishment or injury). "Child Abuse" also means the neglect of a child or abuse in out-of-home care. "Child Abuse" does not mean a mutual affray between minors and does not include any injury caused by reasonable and necessary force used by a peace officer to quell a disturbance threatening physical injury to persons or damage to property, to prevent physical injury or property damage, for purposes of self defense, to obtain possession of weapons or other dangerous objects within control of a child, or apprehend an escapee. [NOTE: State codes may vary.)

## Reporting

All mental health professionals are legally mandated to report when there is "reasonable suspicion" of child abuse in the home or in any other setting. The incident does not have to be observed and does not need to be more than once. When you are employed by an agency that is legally mandated to report, you must sign a statement that you are aware of the reporting requirement and are agreeable to comply. For example, in California, if you suspect child abuse, you must phone a child protective agency right away and file a written report within 36 hours. "Child protective agency" means a police or sheriff's department, a county probation department, or a county welfare department. It does not include a school district police or security department.

California Penal Code. 11165.9 defines a Child Protective Agency as:

> a police or sheriff's department, a county probation department, or a county welfare department. It does not include a school district police or security department.

*Types of Abuse*
- Sexual
- Neglect
- Physical
- Sexual
- Sexual exploitation
- Sexual assault
- Unjustifiable punishment
- Physical corporal punishment

**Sexual abuse** does occur frequently and does form the basis of a very large portion of child and adult psychopathology, with most abuse coming from adults who are trusted, usually parents and adult caretakers. Most incest participants are afraid and unwilling to take part in therapy because of shame, guilt, and the desire to deny or conceal the act. Included in sexual abuse are: rape, oral copulation, incest, child molestation (fondling), sodomy, penetration of genital or anal opening by a foreign object, lewd or lascivious acts–under age 14 (e.g., adult masturbating or exposing self to child).

**Neglect** includes failure to thrive, severe malnutrition, failure to provide medical care, food, shelter, and neglect resulting in injury or death (leaving infant or child alone in car or bathtub).

**Physical abuse** is defined as injury inflicted by other than accidental means:
- If spanking results in bruises, cuts, welts.
- If object is used (such as a belt).
- If discipline is out of control.
- Physical abuse becomes willful cruelty or unjustifiable punishment if it contributes to child's suffering mentally, physically, or endangers the life of the child.

Physical abuse can be described as:
- Mild (a few bruises, cuts, welts, etc.).
- Moderate (single fracture, minor burn, many bruises).
- Severe (many fractures, CNS injury, abdominal injury, large burns, (life-threatening abuse), and finally, death.

**Sexual exploitation:** When using minors to take part in obscene acts (prostitution, modeling, acting) for photography or commercial purposes, film processors are mandated child abuse reporters. In general, for treatment purposes, child abuse and neglect can be defined in terms of the degree to which a parent uses aversive or inappropriate control strategies with his or her child and/or fails to provide minimal standards of care giving and nurturance.

There is a common pattern of parent-child relationship usually associated with child abuse. These factors include:

- The family has broken down or apart.

- The parents feel isolated, having no one to lean on in time of need.
- The abusive act is generated by some form of crisis, real or imagined.
- The spouse is absent, cooperative with the abuse, or fails to provide emotional support for the marital partner.
- The parent unrealistically expects the child to gratify his own dependency needs. The child is seen as different from other children.

## Behavioral Signs of Child Sexual Abuse

In the home and at school, the presence of some of these signs may indicate child abuse and may warrant questioning the child:

- Grades drop and increased problems with concentration.
- Behavior is either overly compliant or child is acting out aggressively.
- Difficulty making friends and relating to peers.
- Inappropriate sexual play, either with self, toys, or peers.
- Sexually aggressive with others and hints about sex.
- Very advanced level of understanding about sexual behavior, but inappropriate for age.
- Doesn't participate in school and social events.
- Few school absences and arrives at school early and stays late.
- Lacks trust of others, especially with significant others.
- Child runs away from home, usually more than once.
- Sleep disturbances.
- Expresses suicidal feelings and being depressed – may attempt suicide
- Behavior regresses.
- Child withdraws from social contact, becomes listless.
- The victim of incest, particularly, may become very compliant.

## Behavioral Signs of Neglected and Battered Children in the Hospital

- Cries very little, or cries hopelessly when being examined or treated.
- Doesn't look to parents for comforting, shows no expectation of comfort.
- Cautious about physical touch from parents or others.
- Shows less fear of the admission process than other children.
- Shows apprehension when adults approach other children and when other children cry.
- Hypervigilant for signs of danger.
- Constantly asking questions: "What happens next?" "When am I going home?" "Will you bring me extra dessert?" "Will you be letting me stay up longer him?"

Generally, neglected and battered children go through life feeling that they are all alone and must face danger by themselves. Children who have been cared for look to their parents for safety.

# Drug Abuse and Addiction in Youth

In the 1999 *Sixth Triennial Report to Congress* on drug use, it is clear that we are making progress on understanding the consequences of illicit drug use through research supported by NIDA, the National Institute on Drug Abuse. We now understand clearly that drug addiction is a chronic, relapsing, treatable brain disease, and we have seen that both behavioral and pharmacological treatments reduce drug use, crime and delinquency, and the spread of HIV/AIDS and other infectious diseases that are associated with drug use and addiction. Scientists have identified neural circuits that subsume the actions of every known drug of abuse, and they have specified common pathways that are affected by almost all such drugs. We have learned more about how an individual's external milieu can affect brain function and, therefore, the addiction process.

A significant breakthrough has been the identification of areas of the brain that are specifically involved in the phenomenon of craving, which is probably the most important factor that can lead to a relapse. NIDA's research shows that that there is a continued high rate of drug use among all groups, but there are indications that drug use is leveling off, particularly among younger age groups (e.g., eighth graders), and that the use of certain drugs among younger age groups may finally be decreasing. In 1999, about 14.8 million Americans over age 12 were current users of illicit drugs (once during month prior to interview). About 3.5 million were dependent on illicit drugs; an additional 8.2 million were dependent on alcohol.

## Tobacco

The use of tobacco products may be the Nation's most critical public health problem, largely because of the addictive properties of nicotine, a major component of tobacco.

In 1997, approximately 71% of the population age 12 or older had tried a few puffs of a cigarette some time in their lives. Cigarette smoking is more common in southern and north central states than in the Northeast or West and more common in non-metropolitan areas. Tobacco is the leading preventable cause of death in the United States.

## Inhalant Use (Commonly known as "huffing")

The highest current use is by 12–17 year olds. In a study in 1997 (Monitoring the Future Study), more than one-fifth of eighth graders had used inhalants at least once in his/her lifetime. In 1999 there were an estimated one million new inhalant users, according to the National Institute of Mental Health, an increase from 10.9 per 1000 potential users to 29 per 1000. Inhalants are most commonly used by adolescents in their early teens, with usage gradually declining with age. Abuse is more common among all socioeconomic levels of American youth than is typically recognized by parents and the general public.

A major roadblock is the ready availability of products that can be inhaled. They are cheap and can be purchased legally as solvents, gases, and nitrites and are inhaled through the nose or mouth, sometimes through a sock or plastic bag which can significantly limit available oxygen in the air and can cause the individual to stop breathing. Common inhalants used by huffers are adhesives, permanent felt tip markers, lighter fluid, spray paint, gasoline, paint thinners, 'white-out', aerosols, butane and flurocarbons from air conditioners.

The National Inhalant Prevention Coalition says that parents can look for these signs:

• Paints or stains on body or clothing
• Spots or sores around the mouth
• Red or runny eyes or nose

- Chemical odor on the breath
- Drunk, dazed or dizzy appearance
- Nausea, loss of appetite

## Hallucinogens

The two most commonly abused are PCP (phencyclidine) and LSD (lysergic acid diethylamide), also known as "acid." In 1997 nearly 10% of the population age 12 and older reported use of hallucinogens at least once during their lifetime. Most users are young, suburban, and middle class. LSD is used by swallowing and absorbing through mouth tissues. PCP (angel dust, boat hog, love boat, peace pill) is injected, swallowed, and smoked. Other hallucinogens are mescaline (buttons, cactus), which is smoked and swallowed, and psilocybin (magic, mushroom, shrooms, purple passion), which is swallowed. Common effects from the hallucinogens are altered states of perception and feeling, nausea/chronic mental disorders, and persisting perception disorder (flashbacks). Symptoms would be beady eyes, nervousness, laughing, crying, personality changes. User sees, smells, and hears color.

## Anabolic Steroids

These are synthetic derivatives of testosterone that promote growth of skeletal muscle and increase lean body mass. Among the class of 1997, 2.4% of high school seniors had used anabolic steroids at least once in their lifetimes. The steroids are injected, swallowed, and applied to the skin. The effects are a premature stoppage of growth (in adolescents), hypertension, hostility and aggression, reduced sperm production, liver cysts, cancer, and blood clotting. In females, menstrual irregularities, development of beard, and other masculine qualities occur in addition to some of the others. Some steroids are: Anadrol, Oxandrin, Durabolin, Depo-Testosterone, Equipoise, "roids," and "juice." There is no intoxicating effect.

## Marijuana

This is the most commonly used illegal drug. Approximately 80% of current illicit drug users are marijuana or hashish users. After 6 years of steady increase, in 1997 marijuana use remained level among eighth graders. The rate decelerated among tenth graders, and for the first time in 6 years, eighth graders reported an increase in disapproval of marijuana. Marijuana-related emergency-room admissions continue to increase. In many US cities, marijuana now exceeds cocaine as the drug most frequently detected by urinalysis among arrested males; use is higher for juveniles than for adults. Marijuana is swallowed, smoked, and eaten and produces euphoria, slowed thinking and reaction time, confusion, impaired balance and coordination, cough, frequent respiratory infections, impaired memory and learning, increased heart rate, anxiety, panic attacks, tolerance, and addiction. Marijuana is stored in the fatty tissues and can remain in the body for 30 days. Common names are: "blunt," "dope," "grass," "joints," "pot," "weed," "reefer," "Mary Jane," "skunk," and "sinsemilla."

## Cocaine

Cocaine use seems to be leveling off among the general population but, as in the past, the rate of current cocaine use in 1997 was highest among those ages 18 – 25 years (1.2%). Rate of use for kids ages 12–17 years was 1%. Cocaine can be injected, smoked, or snorted and causes increased temperature, chest pain, respiratory failure, nausea, abdominal pain, strokes, seizures, headaches, and malnutrition. Other names are: "blow," "bump," "C," "candy," "Charlie," "coke," "crack," "flake," "rock," "snow," and "toot."

## Amphetamines

The use of methamphetamines is a serious and growing problem. The drug has a high potential for abuse and dependence, and because its mood elevating effects can vary in intensity from a few minutes to many hours—depending on the route of administration and dosage—users escalate the frequency and the size of doses to maintain their "high." Amphetamines can be injected, swallowed, smoked, and snorted. Effects from methamphetamine use include aggression, violence, psychotic behavior, memory loss, cardiac and neurological damage, impaired memory and learning, tolerance, and addiction. Names include: Desoxyn, "chalk," "crystal," "fire," "glass," "go-fast," "ice," "meth," and "speed." Among twelfth graders, use was 2.3% in 1997, which remained constant after increasing the previous 4 years.

## Heroin (Opioid)

The conservatively estimated number of heroin users was 68,000 in 1993 compared to 325,000 in 1997. The rates of heroin use in the student population remain quite low, but they have risen significantly among eighth, tenth, and twelfth graders. Snorting or smoking heroin rather than injecting it has played a role in its increased use. Despite this increase, in the past 2 years more students have been reporting heroin use as dangerous. Higher quality and lower priced heroin is available nationwide and is injected, smoked, and snorted. Common names are "brown sugar," "dope," " horse," "H," "junk," "skag," "skunk," "smack," and "white horse."

## MDMA (methylenedioxymethamphetamine): Ecstasy

Abuse of MDMA (ecstasy) has become more widespread in cities across the country. In Boston, MDMA was the most frequently mentioned drug in telephone calls to the Poison Control Center during the first three quarters of the year 2000. Ecstasy is being used in a variety of recreational and social settings, in addition to raves, by a wide variety of age groups. Emergency room reports showed that marijuana abuse in combination with MDMA increased from 8 mentions in 1990 to 796 in 1999.

MDMA injures brain neurons that are critical to regulating mood, emotion, learning, memory, sleep, and pain. It causes mild hallucinogenic effects, increased tactile sensitivity, empathic feelings, hyperthermia, impaired memory and learning. The drug is swallowed and goes by the names: "DOB," "DOM," "Adam," "clarity," "ecstasy," "Eve," "lover's speed," "peace," "STP," "X," and "XTC." It is commonly used in situations of "date rape."

## Emerging Prescription Drugs

Several legal prescription drugs were emerging as drugs of abuse in 1999. These include clonazepam (benzodiazepine) and the controlled substances hydrocodone (Lorcet, Lortab, Vicodin), hydromorphone (Dilaudid), and oxycodone (Percodan, Percocet). The most widely used is hydrocodone. Emergency room mentions of this drug has increased from 6,115 in 1993 to 14,639 in 1999, and combined use with marijuana or hashish increased from 8 in 1990 to 840 in 1999. In some areas, hydromorphone and oxycodone pills are substituted for heroin by heroin abusers. In addition, barbiturates, benzodiazepines, methylphenidate (Ritalin), codeine, methaqualone (Quaalude).

# Diagnosis and Treatment of Drug- and Alcohol-Addicted Youth

Parents, teachers, and family members are usually the ones who will assist the drug-abusing youth in getting help, or treatment. Most often, help is not wanted by the child, but with love, support, legal influence, societal pressure, and determination, the child can be treated in a residential treatment program where he/she will receive a combination of behavioral therapy and pharmacotherapy. The mode of treatment depends on whether the disorder is abuse or addiction. In a few cases of beginning drug abuse, private counseling, parental guidance, and support meetings such as Al-A-Teen, can assist the youth with abstinence. Because of drug cravings, it's very difficult for the child to give up his or her drug of choice while remaining in the same home and community environment. Substance abuse disorders mask or induce many other psychiatric symptoms such as anxiety, psychosis, mood changes, and sleep problems, so the importance of taking a good drug history is vital.

*Table 11-1. Drugs Used by Children and Adolescents*

| Needs | | Desired Effects |
|---|---|---|
| | Through use of Drugs and Alcohol | |
| **These unmet needs:** | > | **Can lead to:** |
| To be stimulated | > | Increased energy |
| To satisfy curiosity | > | New experiences |
| To be accepted | > | To "fit in" with peers |
| To feel confident, loved, respected | > | Security, recognition |
| To feel excited, challenged | > | Relief of boredom |
| To be able to escape from problems, both physical and mental | > | Relief of tension, pain, and worries |
| To have a sense of values or self | > | Making life easier to live, with lowered standards |
| To have control, be in charge | > | Freedom to be own authority figure |
| Physical satisfaction | > | Freedom to express with less inhibitions |
| To feel unique | > | Sense of importance |
| To be able to communicate | > | Freedom to say what you want without worry |
| To be like other family members | > | Status, acceptance, support |

## Child to Staff Relationship

The health care provider who works with children has many stressors, especially because of the many feelings that are generated in the children. Our own parental attitudes are stimulated at work, whether due to our need to love and protect or just to be directive and authoritative. When these attitudes and feelings are provoked, there is always the possibility that the staff may mix up the boundaries of the professional relationship and that of a parent relationship, thereby endangering the therapeutic environment. The following list will serve as warning signs that the therapeutic relationship is endangered. Staff should be open to examining their own behavior and accepting feedback from members if they are observing this happening.

### Twelve Warning Signs in the Child/Staff Relationship
1.  You really don't think of the child as a client.
2.  You are spending your "off" hours either in visiting the client or taking him special gifts and favors.
3.  When you communicate with your peers about your client you only tell the good things about the child's behavior.
4.  You receive phone calls, letters, etc., from the child.
5.  If you are on the evening shift in the hospital and the child is allowed to stay up until you go off duty.
6.  You believe that you are the only person that understands this child.
7.  When someone questions your interactions with the child, you become defensive and guarded.
8.  You blame the family for all the child's problems and believe you could have prevented them, or you believe that the child can't be helped.
9.  You have developed such a "bond" with the child that he/she can be very open with you, especially in light and superficial ways—the relationship can even have sexual overtones—but with other staff the child is guarded, defensive, and avoiding.
10. You are spending far too much time with the child.
11. You keep secrets with the child, not reporting some of the information.
12. This child is "your" patient or client and "yours" alone.

## Grief, Loss, Dying (See also Table 9-2.)

### Development of a Child's Concept of Death:
Development of a child's concept of death:
- Infant - no concept of death
- Toddler - cannot comprehend the concept of death. Child fears separation and develops anxiety due to changes in routine
- Preschooler - no real understanding of the meaning of death. May interpret loss as a punishment for real or imagined wrongdoings
- School-age child - conceptually understands death as the cessation of life. He fears dying.

Elisabeth Kubler-Ross is well known for her work with terminally ill patients. Her book *On Death and Dying* was written after years of research. She and her associates interviewed hundreds of dying patients. The ages were from 16 to 96 years. Almost all socioeconomic levels were represented. The majority were of Judeo-Christian background. Muslims, Hindus, and atheists were included. Despite differences in cultural or religious backgrounds, the terminally ill patients did not vary in their basic needs. Their rituals sometimes differed. Dr. Kubler-Ross divided the pattern of behaviors of dying patients into five distinctive stages. Much of the literature on grieving lacks scientific data, but emphasis is placed on clinical examples and Kubler-Ross's stage of grieving, which follows:

*Kubler-Ross Stages of Grieving. (Remember acronym DABDA)*
- The first stage is **denial**. Even when he has suspected the worst, the patient will not lose hope that there has been some mistake in the diagnosis.
- The second stage is **anger**. The patient releases his anger in all directions and may take it out on caregivers.
- The third stage is **bargaining**. He bargains with God for time.
- The fourth stage is **depression**. Sometimes this is called anticipatory grief.
- The final stage is **acceptance**. This one is not always reached.
  - The patient may seem to have also reached a state of vigilance.
  - Stress level declines from a persistently strong anxiety (hypervigilance) to a moderate intermediate range.
  - The time that patients put their world in order, put their will in order.
  - Proceed to say "good-byes" to family and friends. May appear withdrawn and/or disinterested as family continues to visit and they must say "good-bye" over and over.

*Personal Dynamics of Grieving*
**Shock:** Anesthetized against the overwhelming loss. Not comprehending and not able to face the full magnitude of it.

**Emotional Release:** Beginning to realize how dreadful the loss is. Venting or releasing these feelings is better than trying to repress them.

**Depression, Loneliness, and Utter Isolation:** Feeling of "no help for me." Down in the depths of despair. Should know this is a normal feeling. Aided by expressed concern.

**Physical Symptoms of Distress:** Ill with symptoms related to the loss. Best help is to understand the grief process.

**Panic:** Convinced "something is wrong with me" as a person, can concentrate on little else. May fear they're losing their minds. Best help is to make clear that others feel the same way.

**Guilt Feelings:** May recall own past neglect, mistreatment, or wrong to the deceased. Wrongs may be imaginary, real, or exaggerated, but they may be real wrongs with real guilt. Confession and unburdening of real guilt gives best relief. Guilt feelings are frequent among family and friends in cases of suicide.

*Hostility:* Hostile expressions toward those who "caused" the loss are common. Some hostilities are normal, but not to be encouraged. Often expressed after cases of murder.

*Inability to Renew Normal Activities:* Cannot get back to "business as usual" and must bear loss alone, since others are back to their normal activities. Needs encouragement to face new realities, not to be sheltered from them.

*Gradually Overcoming Grief:* Emotional balance returns little by little, like healing of a physical wound. Healing rate varies with the individual.

*Readjustment to the New Realities:* Not "old self again" because there is a new situation. Is stronger, deeper, and better for having faced and overcome the disaster.

## Nursing Considerations
- Be source of support for patient and family.
- Recognize the stages of grieving.
- Assess child's understanding of death.
- Answer questions truthfully and in simple terms.
- Allow child/family to express feelings openly.
- Assist child/family through the grieving process and allow family to participate in child's care as much as possible.
- Utilize multidisciplinary approach to planning care of child.

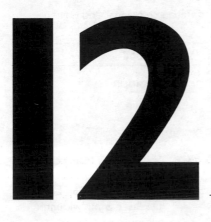

# Review of Psychopharmacotherapy for Children and Adolescents

Over the past two decades, treating childhood mental disorders with psychoactive drugs has become more complex and accepted as an alternative style of treatment. Many drugs produce general and symptom-specific changes in behavior, and clinicians need to be familiar with the differences between drug responses in children vs. drug responses in adolescents. For example, the liver's metabolism in pre-pubertal children is nearly twice that of postpubescent adolescents and consequently reduces the half-life of many psychoactive medications, including tricyclic antidepressants, pemoline, and antipsychotics. Also, prepubescent children have a lower concentration of serum proteins, so they will have a higher free concentration of drugs that are highly protein bound. This would call for administering medications in divided doses and then, after puberty, moving to one dose at night. An interesting fact about adolescent males is that they are especially subject to EPSs with high potency antipsychotics such as Haldol and should receive an anticholinergic as a protection.

There are several classes of drugs used in treating children and adolescents. They are outlined as follows with recommended range of dosage:

## Stimulants
**Uses:** Primarily in adolescent psychiatry to treat attention deficit hyperactivity disorder (ADHD).

**Dosage:** See Table 12-1

**Side effects:** Insomnia, stomach and head aches, loss of appetite, temporary growth suppression. Tics, both vocal and motor, may occur over time. May get tics with some stimulants and not others. This can be resolved by discontinuing the medication. In high doses, can cause a transient paranoid psychosis in younger children. Studies have shown a 5% loss of height with chronic administration. Routine monitoring of height, weight, blood pressure, pulse, lab screening for blood count and liver function recommended. With Cylert use, there has been a 3% incidence of chemical hepatitis, suggesting need for liver function test every 6 months. Routine screening for emergent tics is recommended.

*Table 12-1. Selected Stimulants Used in Adolescent Psychotherapy*

| Medication | Dosage | Titration |
|---|---|---|
| Adderall<br>Adderall XR<br>Dexedrine<br>(dextroamphetamine sulfate) | *Ages 3–5 yrs:* 2.5 mg, PO, qd<br>*Ages 6 and up:* 5 mg, divided in 12 doses, PO, qd | *Ages 3–5 yrs:* May increase dose by 2.5 mg each week. *Ages 6 and up:* Can be increased 5 mg/wk until optimum results are achieved. Maximum dose 40 mg qd |

## Tricyclic Antidepressants

**Uses:** Commonly prescribed for ADHD, enuresis, dysthymia, major depression, anxiety disorders, bulimia, phobias, and conduct disorders.

**Dosage:** (See also Table 12-2.) Typical dosages of these tricyclic antidepressants in pre-pubertal children range up to 5 mg/kg/per day, usually given in 2–3 divided doses.

**Side Effects:** Blurry, dry mouth, constipation, urinary retention, sedation, anticholinergic effects, sometimes combined with cardiovascular abnormalities, skin rashes, seizure risk increased. Norpramin is most lethal in overdose and is given with high risk to pre-pubertal children. A baseline EKG is recommended when on tricyclics, and blood levels are needed at regular intervals.

## Other Antidepressants:

Mao-monoamine oxidase inhibitors (MAOIs)
• Sometimes used to treat depressed adolescents.
• Should not be started sooner than two weeks after treatment with a tricyclic antidepressant or four weeks after trying Prozac.

Prozac (fluoxetine)
• Helpful in treating depression, ADHD, OCD, and phobias.
• Dosage: from 5–80 mg/day; relatively safe in overdose–used with adolescents.
• Side effects include onset insomnia, restlessness. Can be given Trazadone to relieve insomnia.

Wellbutrin (bupropion)
• Role in treating adolescents is unclear; should not be used to treat bulimia—has been used with ADHD and depression.
• Dosage: from 225–300 mg/day in 3 doses.
• Side effects are mild but lowers seizure threshold.

Trazadone (desyrel)
- Used in sedation; sometimes used with mental retardation or autistic disorder to improve sleep patterns and reduce daytime outbursts.
- Dosage: from 50–600 mg/day in 1–3 doses.
- Side effects are mild, except for sedation.

Zoloft (serotonin uptake inhibits, can produce ADHD symptoms)
Paxil (sometimes has more side effects)
Luvox (especially for OCD)

## Anti-Manic

Lithium
- Can be effective for treating bipolar affective disorder, may reduce aggressive outbursts. Not beneficial for treating ADHD; not proven effective in treating adolescent depression.
- Dosage: for pre-pubertal school-aged children, the dosage will be from 600 mg/day to 500 mg/day depending on weight of the child. Three doses a day are advised, with the morning and noon doses being the same, and the evening dose being twice the amount (e.g., 150 mg at 8 a.m., same at noon, and 300 mg at 6 p.m.).
- Side effects include nausea, headache, fine tremor, thirst, polyuria, loose stools.
- Signs of toxicity: vomiting, diarrhea, sleepiness, shaking, slurred speech, dizziness.
- Because there is a risk of birth defects with Lithium treatment, it should be used with caution for females who may become pregnant.
- Regular testing of chemical and hormonal blood levels should be done with Lithium treatment.

Depokote and Tegretol (fewer side effects)

## Antianxiety Agents

Antianxiety agents are used in children and adolescents particularly to treat separation anxiety and obsessive- compulsive disorder. One common symptom of separation anxiety disorder is school refusal.

Tofranil (imipramine)
- Especially useful for school phobia and separation disorder.
- Dosages:
  - For school phobia, it is recommended for ages 6–8 to start on a dose of 10 mg at hs.
  - For older children, 25 mg at bedtime; the dose can be raised 10–50 mg/wk, depending on age. Maximum dose is 3.5 mg/kg/day.
  - For separation anxiety, 25–50 mg/day but may need 75 mg/day if school avoidance is a symptom. Rarely continued for more than 3 months. Behavior improvement usually occurs within the first 2 weeks.
- Side effects include drowsiness and dry mouth.
- Some relapses have occurred after complete remission of symptoms.

Anafranil (clomipramine)
- Effective for controlling symptoms of obsessive compulsive disorder in children and adolescents. Common symptoms are repetitive thoughts of violence, contamination,

or doubt and ritualistic actions involving hand washing, counting, checking, or touching. One study indicated that patients with obsessions responded better than those with compulsions.
* Dosage: range from 100–250 mg/day
* Side effects include tremor, dry mouth, dizziness, constipation, acute dyskinesia, and occasional weight gain.

Benzodiazepines such as Klonopin, Xanax
* Risks for abuse and dependence, sedation, withdrawal symptoms, and disinhibition of impulsive or aggressive behaviors.

Prozac (fluoxetine)
* Sometimes useful when patient cannot tolerate Anafranil.
* Dosage: to treat OCD, the dose usually has to be increased over the dosage needed for depression. Many additional studies of Prozac in treating adolescents are needed before effectiveness is really proven. So far, Anafranil and Prozac are believed to work in about 50% of cases.

## Neuroleptics

Used when aggression is the primary target of behavior, such as hyperactivity, autism, and conduct disorders. Prescribed only when absolutely necessary because neuroleptics have a high risk of side effects. They can cause cognitive and academic impairment. The following drugs are the most commonly prescribed neuroleptics for severe conduct problems:

Mellaril (thioridazine)
* Has been reported to have a favorable effect on seizure reduction. Can be used with epileptic children with behavior disorders.
* Dosage: 10–200 mg/day for children under 12.
* Side effects are frequent and severe: drowsiness, enuresis, increased appetite, mild dry mouth, stomach ache, nausea, vomiting, nosebleeds, tremor, orthostatic hypotension.

Haldol (haloperidol)
* Dosage: effective in .25–16 mg dose/day.
* Side Effects include drowsiness, nausea, ataxia, slurred speech, weight gain, EPSs.

Thorazine (chlorpromazine)
* Dosage: give in same dose as in Mellaril.
* Side effects include skin reactions, diarrhea, upset stomach, blurred vision, dry mouth, constipation and urinary retention.

Risperdol (early antipsychotic, less EPS)

## Psychotropics or Antipsychotics

These are used for a variety of reasons in adolescent psychiatry. They can be used as tranquilizers and can reduce disorganized uncontrolled behavior. Low does may enhance performance in some adolescent autistic disorders. Dosages for adolescents usually are similar to adult doses. Control motor and vocal tics associated with Tourette syndrome.

Haldol (haloperidol)
- Drug of first choice for Tourette syndrome.
- Dosage: very effective for children in low dosage—25–0.5 mg/day and gradually increased to an average daily dose of 3–4 mg/day.
- Side effects include drowsiness, nausea, ataxia, slurred speech, weight gain, EPRs (see above).

Orap (pimozide)
- Both Haldol and Orap are potent D2 receptor blockers and are effective in treating motor and vocal tics of Tourette syndrome.
- Dosage: usually started at 1 mg/day and gradually increased to 6–10 mg/day (0.2 mg/kg/day) Can be given once a day.
- Side effects: can have an adverse effect on heart function. EKG should be done first to establish a baseline.

## Antihypertensive

Catapres (clonidine)
- Uses: Considered to be effective with Tourette syndrome by controlling the associated symptoms of hyperactivity and inattentiveness
- Dosage: Initially small, .05 mg increased over several weeks to 0.15–0.30 mg in small doses 3–4 times/day. It has a slower onset of action than Haldol and could take 3 or more weeks to show improvement. Available in long-acting patch. Side effects include marked sedation, impaired cognition, dry mouth, sensitivity of eyes to light, bradycardia, hypotension, dizziness, irritability, nightmares, insomnia, and postural hypotension. When withdrawing the drug, do it gradually over 10 days to prevent hypertension.

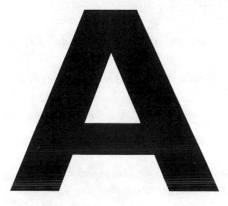

# Appendix A—
## Bibliography

American Nurses Association. (2002). *Code of Ethics for nurses with interpretive statements.* Silver Spring, MD: Author.

American Nurses Association (2004). *Nursing: Scope and Standards of Practice,* 2nd Ed., Silver Spring, MD: Author.

American Nurses Association (2004). *Nursing's Social Policy Statement,* 2nd Ed., Silver Spring, MD: Author.

American Nurses Association. (1993). *Position statement on registered nurse utilization of unlicensed assistive personnel.* Washington, DC: Author.

American Nurses Association. (2000). *Scope & standards of psychiatric-mental health nursing practice.* Washington, DC: Author.

American Psychiatric Association. *Diagnostic and Statistical Manual of Mental Disorders, (DSM-IV-TR),* 4th ed. Washington DC: APA, 2000.

Barkley, R.A. (1981). *Hyperactive children: a handbook for diagnosis and treatment.* New York: Guilford Press

Bartle, J. (2000). Clinical supervision: Its place within the quality agenda. *Nursing Management, 7*(5), 30–33.

Beck, A., Rush, A. J., Shaw, B., & Emery, G. (1979). *Cognitive therapy of depression.* New York: Guilford Press.

Bellenir, K. (Ed.). (2005). *Mental Health Disorders Sourcebook, 3rd Ed.* Detroit: Omnigraphics.

Benner, P. (1984). *From novice to expert: excellence & power in clinical nursing practice.* Menlo Park, CA: Addison-Wesley.

Bick, E. (1968). The experience of the skin in early object-relations. *International Journal of Psychoanalysis, 48*(2), 484–486.

Brent NJ. *Nurses and the Law: A Guide to Principles and Applications,* 2nd ed. Philadelphia: Saunders, 2001.

Caplan, G. (1970). *The theory & practice of mental health consultation.* New York: Basic Books.

Corey, G. (2000). *Theory & practice of group counseling* (5th ed.). Belmont, CA: Wadsworth/Thomson Learning.

Department of Health & Human Services. (1999). *Mental health: A report of the surgeon general.* From www.surgeongeneral.gov.

Drew, C., Logan, D., & Hardman, M. (1994). *Mental Retardation, a life cycle approach* (3rd. ed.) St. Louis: Times Mirror/Mosby

Eliopoulos, C. (1998). Peck's theory on developmental tasks. In *Gerontological nursing.* Philadelphia: Lippincott.

Erikson, E. (1963). *Chldhood & Society.* New York: W. W. Norton.

Erikson, JT., Burton, J., Kaubie, P., Lundberg, L., Charlap-Hyman, A., et. al. (1993). *California laws relating to minors.* Gardena, Ca.: Harcourt Brace Jovanovich Legal and Professional Publications, Inc.

Ewing, J. A. (1984). Detecting alcoholism: The CAGE questionnaire. *Journal of the American Medical Association, 252,* 1905–1907.

Glass, R. (2001). Electroconvulsive therapy: Time to bring it out of the shadows. *Journal of the American Medical Association, 285*(10), 1346–1348.

Glass, R.M. (1999). Treating depression as a recurrent or chronic disease. *Journal of the American Medical Association 201,* 82–84.

Graham M.V., Uphold C.R. (2004). *Clinical Guidelines in Child Health,* 3rd ed. Gainesville FL: Barmarrae Books.

Hamric, A. B., Spross, J. A, Hanson, C. M. (2004). *Advanced Practice Nursing: An Integrative Approach* (3rd ed.). Philadelphia: Saunders.

Heath, H., & Freshwater, D. (2000). Clinical supervision as an emancipatory process: Avoiding inappropriate intent. *Journal of Advanced Nursing, 32*(5), 1298–1306.

Holmes, T., & Rahe, R. (1967). The social readjustment scale. *Journal of Psychosomatic Research, 11,* 213.

Huber, D. (2005). *Leadership & nursing care management* (3rd ed.). Philadelphia: Saunders.

Johnson, D. E. (1980). The Johnson behavioral system model for nursing. In

Jones, A. (1999). Clinical supervision for professional practice. *Nursing Standard, 14*(9), 42–44.

Jones, A. (2001). The influence of professional roles on clinical supervision. *Nursing Standard, 15*(33), 42–45.

Jung, C. (1966). *Two essays on analytical psychology.* Princeton: Princeton University Press.

Kamphaus, R.W. & Frick, P.J. (2005). *Clinical assessment of child and adolescent behavior, 2nd Ed.* Philadelphia: Springer.

Kaplan, H. I., & Sadock, B. J. (2002). *Kaplan and Sadock's Synopsis of psychiatry* (9th ed.). Baltimore, MD: Lippincott, Williams & Wilkins.

Kaufmann, A.S. (1979). *Intelligence testing with the WISC-R.* New York: Wiley Interscience

Keltner N.L., Folks D.G.(2001) *Psychotropic Drugs,* 3rd ed. St. Louis: Mosby.

Kriedler, M., Einsporn, R., Zupancic, M., & Masterson, C. (1999). Group therapy for survivors of childhood sexual abuse who are severely & persistently mentally ill. *Journal of the American Psychiatric Nurses Association, 5*(3), 73–79.[

Kubler-Ross, E. (1969). *On death & dying.* New York: Collier Books, MacMillan.

Kubler-Ross, E. (1987). *AIDS, The ultimate challenge.* New York: Collier Books, MacMillan.

Lewin, K. (1935). A dynamic theory of personality: Selected papers. New York: McGraw-Hill.

Luft, (1984). The johari window: A graphic model of awareness in interpersonal relations. In *Group processes: An introduction to group dynamics* (3rd ed.). Mayfield Publishing Co.

Marek, K. (1989). Outcome measurement in nursing. *Journal of Nursing Quality Assurance, 4*(1), 1–9.

Margolis, S., & Swartz, K. (1999). *Depression & anxiety.* Baltimore, MD: Johns Hopkins Medical Institutions.

Marram, G. (1978). *The group approach in nursing practice.* St. Louis: Mosby.

Mussen, A & Conger, J. (1956). *Child development and personality.* New York: Harper & Brothers.

National Council of State Boards of Nursing. (1990). Concept paper on delegation. Chicago: Author.

National Council of State Boards of Nursing. (1995). Delegation: Concepts & decision-making process. Chicago: Author.

Nicholi, A. (Ed.). (1999). *The Harvard guide to psychiatry* (3rd ed.). Cambridge, MA: Belknap Press of Harvard University Press.

North American Nursing Diagnosis Association. (1999). Nursing diagnoses: Definitions & classification 1999–2000. Philadelphia: Author.

Orem, D. E.: (1980). *Nursing concepts of practice* (2nd ed.). New York: McGraw-Hill.

Peplau, H. E. (1952). *Interpersonal relations in nursing.* New York: G. P. Putnam's Sons.

Polit D.F., Beck C.T. (2003). *Nursing Research: Principles and Methods* (7th ed.). Philadelphia: Lippincott, William and Wilkins.

Proctor, B. (1986). As cited by Fisher, M. (1996). Using reflective practice in clinical supervision. *Professional Nurse, 11*(7), 443–444.

Rother, L. F. (2001). Action stat: Neuroleptic malignant syndrome. *Nursing 2001, 31*(1), 43.

Riehl, J. P., & Roy, C. (Eds.) (1990), *Conceptual models for nursing practice* (2nd ed.). New York: Appleton-Century-Crofts.

Rudorfer, M.V., Henry, M. E., & Sackheim, H.A. (1997). Electroconvulsive therapy. In Tasman, A., Kay, J., & Lieberman, J.A. (Eds.), *Psychiatry* (pp. 1535–1556). Philadelphia: W. B. Saunders.

Selye, H. (1956). *The stress of life.* New York: McGraw-Hill.

Shea, C. A., Pelletier, L. R., Poster, E. C., Stuart, G. W., & Verhey, M. P. (Eds) (1999). *Advanced practice nursing in psychiatric & mental health care.* St. Louis: Mosby.

Shea, S. C. (1998). *Psychiatric interviewing: The art of understanding* (2nd ed.). Philadelphia: Saunders.

Silva, R.R. (Ed.) (2004) *Posttraumatic Stress Disorders in Children and Adolescents Handbook.* New York: W.W. Norton

Sloan, G., White, C. A., & Coit, F. (2000). Cognitive therapy supervision as a framework for clinical supervision in nursing: Using structure to guide discovery. *Journal of Advanced Nursing, 32*(3), 515–524.

Society for Education & Research in Psychiatric-Mental Health Nursing. (1996). Educational preparation for psychiatric-mental health nursing practice. Pensacola, FL: Author.

Stahl, S.M. (2006). *Essential Psychopharmacology: Antipsychotics and Mood Stabilizers.* New York: Cambridge University Press.

Stahl, S. M. (1999). *Psychopharmacology of antipsychotics.* London: Martin Dunitz, Ltd.

Strachey, J. (Ed.) (1959). *Sigmund Freud: Collected Papers (Vol. 5).* New York: Basic Books.

Stuart, G.W., & Laraia, M.T. (Eds.) (2004), *Principles & practice of psychiatric nursing* (8th ed.). St. Louis: Mosby.

Stuart, G., & Sundeen, S. (1995). *Principles & practice of psychiatric nursing.* St. Louis: Mosby.

Talley, S., & Brooke, P. S. (1992). Prescriptive authority for psychiatric clinical specialists: Framing the issues. *Archives of Psychiatric Nursing, 6*(2), p. 72.

Taylor, M. (1987). Self-directed learning: more than meets the observer's eye. In Boud, D., & Griffin, V. (Eds.), *Appreciating adult learning: From the learner's perspective* (pp. 179–196). London: Kogan Page.

U.S. Public Health Service. (1999). The surgeon general's call to action to prevent suicide. Washington, DC.

Von Bertalanffy, L. (1968). *General systems theory: foundations, development, applications.* New York: George Braziller, Inc.

Ward, D. (1999). *AmFAR AIDS handbook The Complete Guide to Understanding HIV and AIDS.* New York: W.W. Norton.

Wetzler, S. & Katz, M.M. (Eds.), (1989). *Contemporary approaches to psychological assessment.* New York: Brunner/Mazel

Wilson, B.A., Shannon, M.T., Shields, K.M. & Stang, C.L. (2007). *Nurse's Drug Guide 2007.* Upper Saddle River, NJ: Pearson-Prentice Hall.

Winnicott, D. W. (1965). The maturational processes & the facilitating environment. London: Hogarth.

Yalom, I. (1983). *Inpatient group therapy.* New York: Basic Books.

Yalom, I. (1985). *The theory & practice of group psychotherapy.* New York: Basic Books.

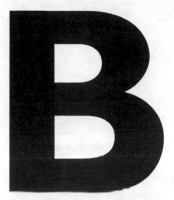

# Appendix B—
## Adult Psychiatric-Mental Health Nursing Review Questions

1. Which disorder is characterized by a chronic, moderately depressed mood and also other symptoms that are similar to, but milder than major depression?
   - a) hypomania
   - b) dysthymia
   - c) Bipolar I disorder
   - d) Bipolar II disorder

2. The activity of which two neurotransmitters in the postsynaptic membrane are elevated by antidepressants?
   - a) dopamine and acetylcholine
   - b) serotonin and dopamine
   - c) serotonin and norepinephrine
   - d) norepinephrine and dopamine

3. Two common symptoms found in individuals with obsessive-compulsive disorder include:
   - a) hypomania and checking behaviors
   - b) checking behaviors and reoccurring thoughts that are difficult to control
   - c) depression and delusional thoughts
   - d) panic attacks and decreased sleep

4. The compulsive behaviors seen in obsessive-compulsive disorder serve to alleviate which symptom in a client?
   - a) anger turned inward
   - b) jealousy
   - c) anxiety
   - d) sadness

5. Which are two medications utilized as mood stabilizers?
   - a) Prozac and a benzodiazepine (Ativan)
   - b) Neuroleptics such as Trilafon or Risperdal and Selective serotonin reuptake inhibitors (SSRIs) such as Celexa and Prozac
   - c) Lithium and anticonvulsants such as Neurontin, Tegretol, and Depakote
   - d) Anticonvulsants (Neurontin, Tegretol, and Depakote) and benzodiazepines (Ativan, Tranxene)

6. Which best describes beliefs that most people would describe as a misrepresentation of reality, or a disorder of thought content?
   a) illusions
   b) delusions
   c) hallucinations
   d) confusion

7. Which neurotransmitter system is most closely associated with schizophrenia and other psychotic disorders?
   a) norepinephrine
   b) serotonin
   c) Substance P
   d) dopamine

8. Which is the most important element in the management of job performance?
   a) Firm disciplinary action
   b) Documentation, including specific dates and times
   c) Maintaining a professional employee/employer distance
   d) Offering acceptable solutions to the employee's problem

9. A 48-year-old woman is admitted on a 72-hour hold because of suicidal ideation. She has a 2-month history of sadness, insomnia, and poor concentration. The symptoms began in the midst of some marital difficulties, but persisted despite an improved home situation. The patient is a sad-appearing, soft-spoken woman without makeup but neatly dressed. She stares at the floor during conversation and shows little expression facially. She has no history of psychiatric disorders.
   Based on the above information, the following can be said about this patient:
   a) Her mood is labile, with a wide range of affect
   b) Her affect is flat
   c) There are no hallucinations or delusions
   d) She is alert and well oriented

10. The ideal phase in the assault cycle to offer prn medication is:
    a) activation phase
    b) early in the escalation phase
    c) crisis phase
    d) recovery phase

11. Helen Singer Kaplan is best known for her work in:
    a) Sex therapy
    b) Group therapy
    c) Crisis intervention
    d) Existential therapy

12. Brevital is:
    a) a short-acting barbiturate
    b) a short-acting muscle relaxant
    c) a slow-acting barbiturate
    d) a slow-acting muscle relaxant

13. On the first day of a mixed-gender group therapy, a woman reveals intimate personal details of her developmental history. The other group members make no comments in support of her. The best explanation for the group's behavior is that:
    a) There are no other women in the group.
    b) The group is struggling to form, which prevents member from responding with support.
    c) The other members do not like her.
    d) The other members' backgrounds and developmental histories are radically different from those of the woman.

14. A group member comments: "I never knew so many people thought like I did." This is an example of which one of Yalom's curative factors?
    a) imitative behavior
    b) universality
    c) corrective reenactment of the primary family group
    d) instillation of hope

15. When the psychiatric nurse asks a client to interpret the saying, "A rolling stone gathers no moss," the nurse is assessing the client's:
    a) abstract thinking
    b) insight
    c) judgment
    d) concentration

16. Which are the physiological effects of prolonged, severe stress on the body?
    a) lowered blood pressure
    b) enlargement of the adrenal cortex and lymphatic structures
    c) decreased cortisol levels
    d) adaptation

17. How do depressants affect the central nervous system in older adult patient?
    a) Depressants have an intensified effect.
    b) Depressants are less effective
    c) There is no difference in effect between adult and geriatric patients.
    d) Compliance is not a problem.

18. A deficiency in dopamine due to blockage of dopamine receptors leads to an imbalance in the:
    a) dopaminergic-cholinergic system
    b) dopaminergic-serotonergic system
    c) cholinergic-serotonergic system
    d) reticular activating system

19. Which statement best defines Lithium?
    a) a complicated metal compound
    b) one of the most effective medications for treatment of mania
    c) a simple metal ion that competes with iron in the blood stream
    d) has a wide therapeutic range and is very seldom toxic

20. The standard dose of which drug is used to approximate the dose equivalent of commonly used antipsychotics?
    a) Prolixin 8 mg
    b) Risperdal 3 mg
    c) Thorazine 100 mg
    d) Clozapine 100 mg

21. Antianxiety agents such as Buspar or Ativan potentiate the therapeutic action which neurotransmitter?
    a) dopamine
    a) acetylcholine
    a) serotonin
    a) GABA

22. Which medication has the potential to induce agranulocytosis or convulsions in the psychotic patient?
    a) risperidone (Risperidone)
    b) clozapine (Clozaril)
    c) haloperidol (Haldol)
    d) quetiapine (Seroquel)

23. The essential feature of neuroleptic malignant syndrome is the development of:
    a) tremors and elevated temperature
    b) changes in level of consciousness
    c) incontinence and muscle rigidity
    d) muscle rigidity and elevated temperature

24. Clients that are addicted to one substance are also addicted to other substances within that same category. This is called:
    a) cross-contamination
    b) cross-tolerance
    c) tolerance
    d) addiction

25. A client comes to the nursing unit with a blood pressure of 180/110 mm Hg, pulse 102 and respirations 20. Hand tremors are present, along with diaphoresis and complaints of anxiety, nervousness. There is a long-standing history of alcohol and cocaine abuse. The client most likely is experiencing:
    a) opiate (narcotic) withdrawal
    b) barbiturate withdrawal
    c) alcohol withdrawal
    d) cocaine withdrawal

26. A client has been drinking 12–16 twelve-ounce cans of beer each day for 7 months. The client states that recently he is requiring more beer to achieve the "high" he is accustomed to. This represents:
    a) tolerance
    b) addiction
    c) withdrawal
    d) intoxication

27. A client comes to the nursing unit with symptoms of hypotension, tachycardia, clammy skin, slow/shallow breathing, depressed levels of consciousness. This client most likely is experiencing:
    a) opiate intoxication
    b) opiate overdose/toxicity
    c) opiate withdrawal
    d) opiate addiction

28. Nursing management of clients with benzodiazepine withdrawal includes:
    a) Administering an opiate, along with comfort measures
    a) Administering a CNS depressant, along with anxiety-producing techniques.
    a) Administering Catapres (clonidine) to block receptor sites
    a) Administering a benzodiazepine along with providing anti-anxiety techniques

29. The following symptoms/behaviors meet the criteria for which DSM-IV-TR diagnosis?
    • Tolerance: a need for markedly increased amounts of the substance to achieve intoxication or desired effect; markedly diminished effect with continued use of the same amount of the substance.
    • Experience of a withdrawal syndrome for the substance.
    • A great deal of time is spent in activities necessary to obtain the substance or recover from its effects.
    • Important social, occupational, or recreational activities are given up or reduced because of substance use.
    a) substance use
    b) substance abuse
    c) substance dependence
    d) substance withdrawal

30. Which neurotransmitter system within the brain precipitates symptoms of anxiety when too little of it is circulating?
    a) norepinephrine
    b) gamma-amino-butyric acid (GABA)
    c) serotonin
    d) opamine

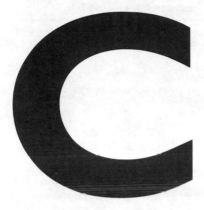

# Appendix C—
Child/Adolescent Psychiatric-
Mental Health Nursing
Study Questions

1. A single parent complains of her 3-year-old son being "out of control" and she "just doesn't know what to do." During your talk you observe son as he interrupts his mother and touches things she told him not to. She further states that the teachers at preschool have no problem with his behavior. Which therapy is best in this situation?
   a) Family therapy because a boy needs his father
   b) Play therapy because the child probably doesn't get to play enough at preschool
   c) Conjoint therapy because the boy and his mother should be treated as equals
   d) Assertion therapy because it can improve the child's behavior through improved parenting skills

2. A mother brings her adolescent daughter to see the psychiatric-mental health nurse so "something" can be done with her, since the mother and daughter don't seem to "understand each other anymore." Using a communications model, the nurse:
   a) States this is a normal phase, a part of the "generation gap," and send them on their way
   b) Sees the daughter alone as this is why the mother has come to you for help
   c) Sees the mother and daughter separately
   d) Requests the entire family attend the next session

3. A family seeks counseling for their son. During an interview session, the mother, sitting next to her son, answered all three questions you have addressed to her son. The behavior observed is an example of:
   a) Poor communication
   b) Enmeshment
   c) Disengagement
   d) A family rule

4. The goal of systems therapy is:
   a) Differentiation of self from the family ego mass
   b) Self-actualization
   c) Increase self-worth
   d) Self-acceptance

5. The processes of Gestalt therapy includes:
   a) Awareness, acceptance, and assimilation
   b) Permission, protection, and potency
   c) Assertion and avoidance
   d) Metaphoric communication

6. According to the psychoanalytic theory, the Electra complex occurs during which of Freud's psychosexual stages of development?
   a) Genital
   b) Latent
   c) Phallic
   d) Anal

7. The expressive therapies include:
   a) Communication, conjoint, dance
   b) Guided imagery, biofeedback, muscle relaxation
   c) Dream interpretation, music, relaxation
   d) Art, music, play

8. The rational application of structured sexual experiences in the treatment of sexual dysfunctions is proposed by:
   a) Gerald Caplan and Karen Horney
   b) Harold Kaplan and Benjamin Sadock
   c) Helen Kaplan and Masters and Johnson
   d) Helen Horney and Masters and Johnson

9. To be diagnosed with encopresis, a child must be:
   a) At least 4 years old or at least an equivalent developmental level
   b) At least 7 years old and suffer from low self-esteem
   c) Having multiple bowel movements every day
   d) Receiving laxatives daily

10. In the past 2 months, an 8-year-old third grader has resisted going to school. She complains of headaches, stomachaches, or other vague discomforts almost every morning and begs her mother to let her stay home. When she is at school, she is anxious and worried. She says she is afraid her house will burn down while she is at school and that no one will tell her about it. These symptoms are suggestive of which disorder?
    a) Generalized anxiety disorder
    b) Separation anxiety disorder
    c) Avoidant personality disorder
    d) Reactive attachment disorder

11. The recommended length of time for a "time out" is:
    a) 5 minutes for preschoolers, 10 minutes for school-age children
    b) 20 minutes regardless of age
    c) 1–2 minutes per year of age
    d) Depends on child's temperament

12. A day care worker is concerned about a 4-year-old because he responds to both caregivers and his parents in a detached, inhibited manner. In addition, he is always hypervigilant and cannot relax and play successfully with other children. The day care worker is also aware that the boy has been in several foster placements due to abuse and neglect. This child most likely suffers from:
    a) Reactive attachment disorder
    b) Attention deficit disorder
    c) Autistic disorder
    d) Separation anxiety disorder

13. A mother tells the pediatrician that her 3-year-old daughter has a habit of repeatedly banging her head on the floor. The mother is worried because this behavior is taking more and more of her daugher's time and she no longer shows an interest in her toys or in playing with her older sister. This child most likely has:
    a) Stereotypic movement disorder
    b) OCD
    c) Simple tic disorder
    d) Autistic disorder

14. In the past 2 years, a 16-year-old has changed her hairstyle and mode of dressing several times. One week she expresses a desire to be a movie actress; the next week, an airline pilot. Sometimes she seems to make mature decisions and at other times seems to regress to childlike behavior. Her parents are distressed. What is the best explanation for the psychiatric mental-health nurse to provide to the parents?
    a) The daughter may be experiencing multiple personality disorder
    b) The daughter needs close observation for development of loose associations
    c) Most probably, the daughter is working through a normal developmental stage of adolescence
    d) It is likely that the daughter has a drug addiction

15. When assessing for potential developmental disabilities in a child, it is important to receive information relating to:
    a) Preferences of colors and shapes
    b) History of pregnancy and delivery and Apgar rating
    c) Child's ability to walk on his or her toes
    d) Child's age at potty training

16. In what areas does the psychicatric-mental health nurse expect to find abnormal development in a child diagnosed with autism?
    a) Gross motor skills, head size, communication
    b) Social skills, communication, behavior
    c) Behavior, fine motor skills, hearing
    d) An obcessive desire to have things constantly changing

17. A 10-year-old girl is referred by her school counselor because she is disruptive, has been fighting and touching boys inappropriately. She speaks English and moved to California from Mexico one year ago when her father died. She lives with her uncle and his 15-year-old son. She has nightmares every night but the uncle says this is normal. This situation most likely involves:
    a) Mental retardation
    b) Drug abuse
    c) Child abuse
    d) V. codes

18. A 16-year-old girl is admitted to the inpatient unit with a tentative diagnosis of schizophrenia. She has episodes of school absenteeism, withdrawal from her friends, and bizarre behavior, including talking to her "keeper." The psychiatric nurse's most appropriate initial response is to:
    a) Encourage the girl to express her thoughts to determine the meaning they have for her.
    b) Tell the girl that her perceptions of reality have become distorted because of her illness.
    b) Ignore the girl's bizarre behavior because it will disappear after she has been given the correct medication.
    b) Acknowledge that the girl's perceptions seem real to her and refocus her attention on a task or activity.

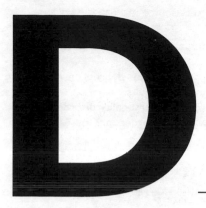

# Appendix D—
## Answers to Adult Psychiatric-Mental Health Nursing Review Questions

1. Which disorder is characterized by a chronic, moderately depressed mood and also other symptoms that are similar to, but milder than major depression?
   a) Incorrect. Hypomania does not have moderate depressed mood, the mood is mildly elevated.
   b) Correct. Dysthymia is a chronic (over 2 years) moderately depressed mood, along with low self-esteem and feelings of helplessness
   c) Incorrect. Bipolar I disorder
   d) Incorrect. Bipolar II disorder

2. The activity of which two neurotransmitters in the postsynaptic membrane are elevated by antidepressants?
   a) Incorrect. Antipsychotics assist in decreasing dopamine; anticholinergics primarily target acetylcholine.
   b) Incorrect. SSRI antidepressants target serotonin, antipsychotics target dopamine.
   c) Correct. SSRIs (antidepressants) target serotonin and SNRIs (antidepressants) target serotonin and norepinephrine.
   d) Incorrect. Norepinepherine is associated with depression but dopamine is not.

3. Two common symptoms found in individuals with obsessive-compulsive disorder include:
   a) Incorrect. Checking behaviors is associated with obsessive-compulsive disorder; however, hypomania is associated with bipolar disorder.
   b) Correct. Both checking behaviors and reoccurring thoughts that are difficult to control are associated with obsessive compulsive disorder.
   c) Incorrect. Depression is part of a mood disorder, and delusional thoughts are associated with a thought disorder, such as schizophrenia.
   d) Incorrect. Panic attacks are associated with panic disorder and decreased sleep is associated with major depression.

4.  The compulsive behaviors seen in obsessive-compulsive disorder serve to alleviate which symptom in a client?
    a) Incorrect. Anger turned inward is a symptom of major depression, as the anger is turned in upon the self and depression results.
    b) Incorrect. Jealousy is associated with narcissistic personality disorder.
    c) Correct. Anxiety is associated with the anxiety disorders and obsessive-compulsive disorder is one of the anxiety disorders.
    d) Incorrect. Sadness is associated with bereavement and or one of the mood disorders.

5.  Which are two medications utilized as mood stabilizers?
    a) Incorrect. Prozac is an antidepressant; Ativan is a central nervous system depressant.
    b) Incorrect. Neuroleptics such as Trilafon or Risperdal are not used as mood stabilizers; selective serotonin reuptake inhibitors (SSRIs) such as Celexa and Prozac assist with elevating mood, but not in stabilizing a manic patient's mood.
    c) Correct. Lithium and anticonvulsants such as Neurontin, Tegretol, and Depakote are used as mood stabilizers.
    d) Incorrect. Anticonvulsants (Neurontin, Tegretol, and Depakote) are mood stabilizers; however, Ativan and Tranxene (both benzodiazepines) are central nervous system depressants.

6.  Which best describes beliefs that most people would describe as a misrepresentation of reality, or a disorder of thought content?
    a) Incorrect. Illusions are distortions of visual perceptions.
    b) Correct. Delusions are beliefs that most people would describe as a misrepresentation of reality.
    c) Incorrect. Hallucinations are either visual, auditory, gustatory, and/or tactile and are not beliefs.
    d) Incorrect. Confusion is a disorientation to reality-based information, such as person, time, and place.

7.  Which neurotransmitter system is most closely associated with schizophrenia and other psychotic disorders?
    a) Incorrect. The norepinephrine system is implicated in depression.
    b) Incorrect. The serotonin system is implicated in depression.
    c) Incorrect. It is unknown what is implicated by the Substance P system.
    d) Correct. The dopaminergic system is implicated in schizophrenia.

8.  Which is the most important element in the management of job performance?
    a) Incorrect. Disciplinary action without solutions will only continue the problem.
    b) Incorrect. Documentation is important, however, it is not the most important.
    c) Incorrect. A strong collegial relationship is encouraged, more so than distance.
    d) Correct. Offering acceptable solutions assists in developing a win-win situation and improves the supervisor/supervisee relationship.

9.  Based on the above information, the following can be said about this patient:
    a) Incorrect. No indication is made of a labile, or wide range of affect.
    b) Correct answer. This patient displayed little expression facially.
    c) Incorrect. No information was given regarding hallucinations/delusions
    d) Incorrect. No information was given as to orientation or alertness.

10. The ideal phase in the assault cycle to offer prn medication is:
    a) The correct answer is a. The activation phase is Phase I of the assault cycle.
    During the activation phase the patient is still able to hear the nurse and can
    make rational decisions. By offering a prn medication at this time, the patient
    can calm down and deescalate. If the behavior is allowed to continue, the
    patient's behavior will escalate, she will not be able to handle additional stimuli,
    and the situation can easily progress to the crisis phase. The crisis phase and
    recovery phase are not the ideal times to administer prn medications.

11. Helen Singer Kaplan is best known for her work in:
    a) Correct.
    b) Incorrect. Group therapy is associated with Yalom
    c) Incorrect. Crisis intervention is associated with Gerald Caplan.
    d) Incorrect. Existential therapy is associated with Fritz Perls.

12. Brevital is:
    a) A is correct. Brevital is a short-acting barbiturate, not a muscle relaxant and
    not long acting.

13. On the first day of a mixed-gender group therapy, a woman reveals intimate
    personal details of her developmental history. The other group members make no
    comments in support of her. The best explanation for the group's behavior is that:
    a) Incorrect. There are women in the group.
    b) Correct. In the beginning stages of group therapy, less personal information
    is shared.
    c) Incorrect. They do no know her yet.
    d) Incorrect. Best answer is group process answer re: stages of group therapy.

14. A group member comments: "I never knew so many people thought like I did." This
    is an example of which one of Yalom's curative factors?
    a) Incorrect. This is when one imitates another's behaviors.
    b) Correct. That we are not alone in our struggles is the healing concept of
    universality
    c) Incorrect. Family group was not reenacted in this scenario, nor is patient
    playing out his or her role in family.
    d) Incorrect. No instillation of hope in this scenario; focus is universality.

15. When the psychiatric nurse asks a client to interpret the saying, "A rolling stone
    gathers no moss," the nurse is assessing the client's:
    a) Abstract thinking is correct.

16. Which are the physiological effects of prolonged, severe stress on the body?
    a) Incorrect. Stress usually increases BP.
    b) Correct.
    c) Incorrect. Stress increases cortisol.
    d) Incorrect. Prolonged severe stress cannot be adapted to indefinitely.

17. How do depressants affect the central nervous system in older adult patient?
    a) Correct. Central nervous system depressants have an intensified effect in the elderly.
    b) Incorrect. Depressants are more effective in the elderly.
    c) Incorrect. There is a difference in effect between adult and geriatric patients' response to depressants.
    d) Incorrect. Compliance with their own medical regimen is a problem in the elderly.

18. A deficiency in dopamine due to blockage of dopamine receptors leads to an imbalance in the:
    a) Correct. The dopamine deficiency leads to an imbalance in the dopaminergic-cholinergic system.
    b) Incorrect. It is the dopaminergic-cholinergic system that is put out of balance when the dopamine receptors are blocked.
    c) Incorrect. It is the dopaminergic-cholinergic system that becomes imbalanced when psychoactive drugs block the dopamine receptors.
    d) Incorrect. Rationale: The reticular activating system is not depressed by neuroleptics.

19. Which statement best defines Lithium?
    a) Incorrect. Lithium is a simple metal ion.
    b) Correct. Lithium is one of the most effective medications for the treatment of mania.
    c) Incorrect. Lithium can cause toxic effects by competing with sodium throughout the body. It does not compete with iron.
    d) Incorrect. Lithium has a narrow therapeutic range and can easily be toxic.

20. The standard dose of which drug is used to approximate the dose equivalent of commonly used antipsychotics?
    a) Incorrect. Prolixin is not the antipsychotic that is used to approximate dose equivalent of commonly used agents.
    b) Incorrect. Risperdal is an atypical and has fewer side effects when compared to Thorazine.
    c) Correct. Thorazine was the first antipsychotic used with success for schizophrenia. Its standard dose, 100 mg, is used to approximate dose equivalents of commonly used agents.
    d) Incorrect. Clozapine is the first atypical antipsychotics. Clozapine 50 mg equals the potency of Thorazine 100 mg.

21. Antianxiety agents such as Buspar or Ativan potentiate the therapeutic action of which neurotransmitter?
    d) D, GABA.

22. Which medication has the potential to induce agranulocytosis or convulsions in the psychotic patient?
    b) B, clozapine.

23. The essential feature of neuroleptic malignant syndrome is the development of:
    d) D, muscle rigidity and elevated temperature.

24. Clients that are addicted to one substance are also addicted to other substances within that same category. This is called:
    a) Incorrect. Cross-contamination is related to the subject of asepsis, not substance abuse/dependency.
    b) Correct answer. Cross-tolerance is when a client is addicted to one substance and is also addicted to other substances within the same drug category.
    c) Incorrect. Tolerance is when an individual requires more of the substance/drug to get the desired effects.
    d) Incorrect. Addiction is physical and/or psychological dependency upon a drug or substance.

25. A client comes to the nursing unit with a blood pressure of 180/110 mm Hg, pulse 102 and respirations 20. Hand tremors are present, along with diaphoresis and complaints of anxiety, nervousness. There is a long-standing history of alcohol and cocaine abuse. The client most likely is experiencing:
    a) A and b are incorrect. There is no information that client was taking any narcotics or barbiturates. The symptoms listed are all symptoms of alcohol withdrawal.
    b) Correct. Symptoms listed are all symptoms of alcohol withdrawal.
    c) Incorrect. Cocaine withdrawal is characterized.

26. A client has been drinking 12–16 twelve-ounce cans of beer each day for 7 months. The client states that recently he is requiring more beer to achieve the "high" he is accustomed to. This represents:
    a) Correct. Tolerance is requiring more of a drug/substance to achieve the desired effect.
    b) Incorrect. Addiction is physical and/or psychological dependency upon a drug or substance.
    c) Incorrect. Withdrawal is the presence of substance-specific symptoms exhibited upon the cessation of a drug/substance.
    d) Incorrect. Intoxication is the ingestion of a large quantity of a drug/substance that produces specific symptoms based on the drug/substance consumed.

27. A client comes to the nursing unit with symptoms of hypotension, tachycardia, clammy skin, slow/shallow breathing, depressed levels of consciousness. This client most likely is experiencing:
    b) B is correct. Opiate overdose/toxicity is characterized by the symptoms listed.

28. Nursing management of clients with benzodiazepine withdrawal includes:
    a) Incorrect. Benzodiazepine w/d requires administration of the same or another benzodiazepine along with comfort measures.
    b) Incorrect. It is more specific to administer a benzodiazepine rather than a "CNS depressant" during benzodiazepine w/d. Also, it is not appropriate to provide anxiety-producing techniques.
    c) Incorrect. Administering Catapres (clonidine) is appropriate in narcotic w/d, not benzodiazepine w/d.
    d) Correct. This is the most specific and appropriate response.

29. The following symptoms/behaviors meet the criteria for which DSM-IV-TR diagnosis?
    a) Incorrect. The symptoms listed are more detrimental to the client than mere substance use.
    b) Incorrect. Substance abuse is characterized by the symptoms listed; however, substance dependence is the most correct answer.
    c) Correct. Substance dependence is most clearly the presence of tolerance, withdrawal syndrome, spending a great deal of time obtaining the substance, and reduction in social activities.
    d) Incorrect. Substance w/d is the presence of substance-specific symptoms after cessation from a drug/substance.

30. Which neurotransmitter system within the brain precipitates symptoms of anxiety when too little of it is circulating?
    a) Incorrect. Too little norepinephrine is associated with depression.
    b) Correct. Too little gamma-amino-butyric acid (GABA) is associated with symptoms of anxiety.
    c) Incorrect. Too little serotonin is associated with symptoms of depression.
    d) Incorrect. Too much dopamine is associated with schizophrenia.

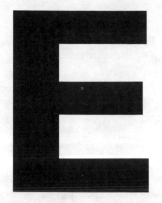

# Appendix E—
Answers to Child/Adolescent Psychiatric-Mental Health Nursing Review Questions

1. d
2. d
3. b
4. a
5. a
6. c
7. d
8. c
9. a
10. b
11. c
12. a
13. a
14. c
15. b
16. b
17. d
18. d

# Index